SUPER
LOW-CARB
SNACKS

Brimming with creative inspiration, how-to projects, and useful information to enrich your everyday life, Quarto Knows is a favorite destination for those pursuing their interests and passions. Visit our site and dig deeper with our books into your area of interest: Quarto Creates, Quarto Cooks, Quarto Homes, Quarto Lives, Quarto Drives, Quarto Explores, Quarto Gifts, or Quarto Kids.

First Published in 2019 by Fair Winds Press, an imprint of The Quarto Group, 100 Cummings Center, Suite 265-D, Beverly, MA 01915, USA.
T (978) 282-9590 F (978) 283-2742 QuartoKnows.com

Fair Winds Press titles are also available at discount for retail, wholesale, promotional, and bulk purchase. For details, contact the Special Sales Manager by email at specialsales@quarto.com or by mail at The Quarto Group, Attn: Special Sales Manager, 100 Cummings Center, Suite 265-D, Beverly, MA 01915, USA.

23 22 21 20 19   1 2 3 4 5

ISBN: 978-1-59233-911-2

Digital edition published in 2019

The content that appears in this book previously appeared in the following books published by Fair Winds Press: *200 Low-Carb, High-Fat Recipes* (2014), by Dana Carpender; *Super Paleo Snacks* (2014), by Landria Voigt; *Sweet and Savory Fat Bombs* (2016), by Martina Slajerova.

Library of Congress Cataloging-in-Publication Data available

Design: Sporto
Cover Images: Martina Slajerova
Page Layout: Sporto
Photography: Martina Slajerova and Landria Voigt

Printed in China

The information in this book is for educational purposes only. It is not intended to replace the advice of a physician or medical practitioner. Please see your health-care provider before beginning any new health program.

SUPER
LOW–CARB
SNACKS

100 Delicious **KETO** and **PALEO** Treats
for Fat Burning and Great Nutrition

Martina Slajerova, Landria Voigt, C.H.H.C., and Dana Carpender

FAIR WINDS

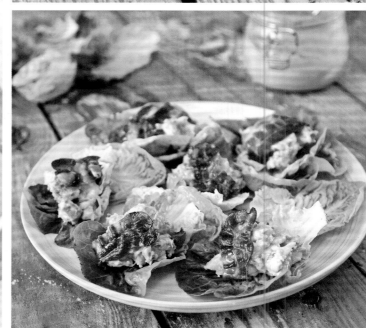

CONTENTS

INTRODUCTION

The Importance of Healthy Snacking

Almost everyone snacks. A 2010 study in the *Journal of Nutrition* found that 24 percent—nearly a quarter—of our total energy intake comes from snacks. For something that contributes to our diet as much as breakfast, lunch, and dinner do, it's somewhat surprising that relatively few people know whether they follow good snacking habits—or even that there is such a thing as a "good snack habit."

Most snacks consumed today skew toward the prepackaged and processed kinds that are high in refined sugar, white flour, gluten, and food coloring while being low in nutrition. Consuming these foods is, in general, bad for you and your health.

This book offers healthy alternatives: one-hundred low-carb, Paleo- and Keto-friendly, whole-food snacks. These snacks will satisfy your between-meals hunger and provide you with the energy you need, whether it's at work or school, on the road, at home, during a workout, or any time. They include:

- "Fat bombs"—high in fat and low in protein and carbohydrates, they're the ideal snacks if you're eating low carb. Choose a fat bomb anytime, such as when you don't have time to cook and need a quick hit of energy or as pre- or post-workout snacks instead of "regular" snacks that are high in carbs.

- Basic nut and seed butters and sugar-free chocolates provide the foundation for healthy snacking. Easy to make, use them in place of peanut butter, in smoothies, as a healthy way to satisfy a sweet tooth, and as the basis for other low-carb recipes.

- Sippable snacks, both hot and cold, are easy to take on the go or enjoyed slowly when you have time to yourself. (Some of these recipes are high in calories, so if calories are important to you, take note and adjust accordingly.)

- An entire chapter devoted to nut-free, dairy-free, and egg-free options in one easy-to-find place. (Note that additional allergy-free recipes can be found throughout the book as denoted by the icons in the "Got Allergens" chart below.)

Got Allergies

If you're concerned about allergens, look for these icons at the top of recipes:

 Dairy-Free

 Egg-Free

 Nut-Free

The Benefits of Snacking

It is important to understand that snacking is not only normal, but it is also an absolutely healthy endeavor, as long as the nutritional value of the snack is beneficial. We snack for many reasons, the primary of which is to stave off hunger in between meals.

Yet snacking provides a number of physical and cognitive perks, too. It can boost cognitive focus throughout the work and school day by helping us maintain blood sugar levels. Our bodies digest whole foods that include fats, proteins, and fiber—such as the ones in this book—at a slower and more consistent rate, and therefore release a steadier stream of glucose to the brain. Conversely, a snack that is high in refined sugar and white flour will spike insulin levels and cause one to be hungrier and less focused in a shorter time. The snacks in this book contain ingredients such as meat, eggs, and nuts that will hold hunger at bay while keeping you tack sharp.

Another benefit of snacking is that it helps prevent overeating at mealtime. There's a difference between "ruining your dinner" and preparing your body with vital nutrients. Sitting down to dinner with that "I'm famished" feeling can lead you to consume more calories than you actually need. In a state of heightened hunger, you tend to eat faster. Numerous studies have shown that individuals who eat slower typically consume fewer calories than their fast-eating peers. Science suggests this is because of a communication lag between the receptors in your stomach and those in your brain—in other words, between having a full stomach and the realization that you're satiated. So by helping quell the feeling of hunger through more consistent engagement of stomach receptors, appropriate pre-meal snacks might actually help you lose weight.

For anyone who works out or plays a sport, preworkout snacks are imperative to optimizing performance. The right balance of protein can help us keep our mind focused and increase endurance by slowing muscle breakdown during activity. Also important is having the right postworkout snacks in your bag. We lose many minerals through the excretion of sweat during exercise, and those minerals need to be replaced quickly so our bodies can work efficiently. With a deficiency of certain minerals, such as magnesium, we may have fatigue, muscle cramps, trouble maintaining blood sugar levels, and a harder time getting oxygen into our muscle cells.

Recognizing When It's Truly Time for a Snack

When you really think about it, what is it to "feel hungry"? The signs are usually much more subtle than a rumbling tummy, which can often be quelled by a glass of water, as many times we mistake thirst for hunger. Is your energy starting to wane? Perhaps your ability to focus on the task at hand is becoming more of a challenge. Are you becoming a bit more irritable? When any of these symptoms start to surface, it's snack time.

This book offers you one hundred deliciously low-carb recipes to choose from, as well as nutritional and allergy-related information, so you can make an informed choice. Need fuel for a road race? At home or on the go? Want to sip your snack? Need a nut-free nosh? *Super Low-Carb Snacks* has you covered.

1

THE BASICS:
Versatile, Homemade Nut Butters and Sugar-Free Chocolates

The Basics

Before you start creating low-carb snacks, including fat bombs, you'll need to make a few simple-to-prepare, basic ingredients, such as nut and seed butters and homemade chocolate. Most nut and seed butters can be kept at room temperature for a few days, and will last for several weeks in a sealed glass jar in the refrigerator. You can also freeze nut and seed butters for 3 to 4 months. Homemade chocolate will keep refrigerated for up to 3 months. The best part is, in addition to being delicious, all these recipes are sugar free.

Almond and Cashew Butter

This delicious spread is a great paleo alternative to peanut butter.

1 cup (150 g /5.3 oz) almonds, blanched or whole

1/3 cup (50 g /1.8 oz) cashews

4 tablespoons (60 ml /2 fl oz) almond oil or macadamia nut oil

Pinch salt (optional)

Seeds from 1 vanilla bean (optional)

1/2 teaspoon ground cinnamon (optional)

1. Preheat the oven to 350°F (175°C, or gas mark 4). Spread the almonds and cashews on a baking sheet and place in the preheated oven for 12 to 15 minutes. Watch carefully to prevent burning. Remove from the oven and cool.

2. In a food processor, pulse the nuts until smooth (or reserve some chopped nuts to add later for a chunkier texture). Depending on your processor, this may take some time. At first, the mixture will be dry. Scrape down the sides several times with a rubber spatula if the mixture sticks.

3. Add the oil. Continue to blend until you reach the desired consistency. The oil makes the butter smoother and more suitable for creating fat bombs. Add the salt and vanilla bean seeds or cinnamon (if using) and pulse to combine. Spoon the butter into a glass container. Seal and store at room temperature for up to 1 week or refrigerate for up to 3 months.

YIELD: about 1 cup (250 g/8.8 oz)

....

NUTRITIONAL FACTS

Per serving (2 tablespoons [1.1 ounce, or 32 g]): total carbs: 5.5 g; fiber: 2.1 g; net carbs: 3.4 g; protein: 5.2 g; fat: 19.4 g; energy: 205 kcal.

Macronutrient ratio: calories from carbs: 6 percent; protein: 10 percent; fat: 84 percent.

Coconut and Pecan Butter

Keep a napkin handy. You'll drool over this cinnamon-spiced nut butter. Made with pecans and coconut, it's perfect for making chocolate treats.

2 cups (150 g/5.3 oz) unsweetened shredded coconut

1 cup (100 g/3.5 oz) pecans

1 teaspoon sugar-free vanilla extract or

½ teaspoon vanilla powder

1 teaspoon ground cinnamon

¼ teaspoon salt

1. In a food processor, combine the coconut, pecans, vanilla, cinnamon, and salt. Pulse until smooth and creamy. Depending on your processor, this may take a few minutes. At first, the mixture will be dry. Scrape down the sides several times with a rubber spatula if the mixture sticks.

2. Spoon the butter into a glass container. Seal and store at room temperature for up to 1 week or refrigerate for up to 3 months.

YIELD: about 1 cup (250 g/8.8 oz)

....

NUTRITIONAL FACTS

Per serving (2 tablespoons [1.1 ounce, or 32g]): total carbs: 6.5 g; fiber: 4.4 g; net carbs: 2.1 g; protein: 5 g; fat: 11.6 g; energy: 154 kcal.

Macronutrient ratio: calories from carbs: 6 percent; protein: 15 percent; fat: 79 percent.

To enhance this butter's flavor, use roasted pecans and coconut: Preheat the oven to 350°F (175°C, or gas mark 4). Spread the coconut and pecans on a baking sheet. Place in the preheated oven and roast for 5 to 8 minutes, or until the coconut is lightly golden. Stir once or twice to prevent burning.

Chocolate-Hazelnut Butter

This healthy, low-carb alternative to Nutella is just the thing for making truffles, and it's also great in smoothies.

1 cup (150 g/5.3 oz) hazelnuts

1 cup (130 g/4.6 oz) macadamia nuts

½ cup (75 g/2.6 oz) almonds

1 bar (100 g/3.5 oz) extra-dark chocolate, 85 percent cacao or more

1 tablespoon (15 g/0.5 oz) coconut oil

1 tablespoon (5 g/0.2 oz) unsweetened cacao powder

1 teaspoon sugar-free vanilla extract or ½ teaspoon vanilla powder

2 tablespoons (20 g/0.7 oz) erythritol or Swerve, powdered

Few drops liquid stevia, to taste (optional)

½ cup (120 ml/4 fl oz) coconut milk or heavy whipping cream (optional)

1. Preheat the oven to 375°F (190°C, or gas mark 5). Spread the hazelnuts, macadamia nuts, and almonds on a baking sheet. Place in the preheated oven and bake for about 10 minutes, or until lightly browned. Remove the nuts from the oven and cool for 15 minutes.

2. Meanwhile, melt the dark chocolate and coconut oil in a double boiler, or heat-proof bowl placed over a small pot filled with 1 cup (235 ml) of boiling water, making sure the water doesn't touch the bottom of the bowl. Stir until melted.

3. Rub the hazelnuts together in your hands to remove the skins. This makes the butter smooth and avoids the bitter taste imparted by the skins. Place all of the nuts into a food processor and pulse until smooth.

4. Add the cacao powder, vanilla, erythritol, and stevia (if using) to the melted chocolate. Pour the mixture into the processor with the nuts and pulse until smooth. If you're using the coconut milk, add it to the processor and pulse again.

5. Transfer the butter to a glass container. Seal and refrigerate for up to 3 months, or 4 weeks if using coconut milk or cream.

YIELD: about 2 cups (500 g/1.1 lbs)

NUTRITIONAL FACTS

Per serving (2 tablespoons [1.1 ounce, or 32 g]): total carbs: 5.9 g; fiber: 2.9 g; net carbs: 3 g; protein: 3.9 g; fat: 18.7 g; energy: 193 kcal.

Macronutrient ratio: calories from carbs: 6 percent; protein: 8 percent; fat: 86 percent.

▶ To powder the erythritol, place it in a clean blender or coffee grinder and pulse until powdery, about 15 to 20 seconds.

Eggnog-Macadamia Butter

Enjoy the flavors of the holiday season all year 'round! This macadamia-based butter is lightly spiced, creamy, and addictive.

2 cups (260 g/9.2 oz) macadamia nuts

1 teaspoon ground nutmeg

1/2 teaspoon sugar-free vanilla extract or 1/4 teaspoon vanilla powder

1/2 teaspoon ground cinnamon

1/2 teaspoon natural rum extract

2 tablespoons (20 g/0.8 oz) erythritol or Swerve, powdered

Few drops liquid stevia, to taste (optional)

In a food processor, combine the macadamia nuts, nutmeg, vanilla, cinnamon, rum extract, and erythritol. Add a few drops of stevia (if using). Process until smooth. The exact amount of time depends on your processor. Spoon the butter into a glass container. Seal and store at room temperature for up to 1 week or refrigerate for up to 3 months.

YIELD: about 1 cups (290 g/10.2 oz)

....

NUTRITIONAL FACTS

Per serving (2 tablespoons [32 g/1.1 oz]): total carbs: 4.6 g; fiber: 2.8 g; net carbs: 1.8 g; protein: 2.3 g; fat: 21.7 g; energy: 209 kcal.

Macronutrient ratio: calories from carbs: 3 percent; protein: 4 percent; fat: 93 percent.

White Chocolate and Macadamia Butter

This recipe combines some of the healthiest high-fat foods in a single jar of goodness: macadamia nuts, coconut butter, and cacao butter. The result? A white chocolate treat that's good for you, too.

1 cup (130 g/4.7 oz) macadamia nuts

½ cup (125 g/4.4 oz) coconut butter

½ cup (110 g/3.9 oz) cacao butter

2 teaspoons sugar-free vanilla extract or 1 teaspoon vanilla powder

¼ cup (40 g/1.4 oz) erythritol or Swerve, powdered

Few drops liquid stevia, to taste (optional)

In a food processor, combine the macadamia nuts, coconut butter, cacao butter, vanilla, and erythritol. Add the stevia (if using), and process until smooth. The exact amount of time depends on your processor. Spoon the butter into a glass container. Seal and store at room temperature for up to 1 week or refrigerate for up to 3 months.

YIELD: about 1 ⅔ cups (410 g/14.5 oz)

....

NUTRITIONAL FACTS

Per serving (2 tablespoons [1.1 ounce, or 32 g]): total carbs: 3.7 g; fiber: 2.4 g; net carbs: 1.3 g; protein: 1.4 g; fat: 21.8 g; energy: 207 kcal.

Macronutrient ratio: calories from carbs: 2 percent; protein: 3 percent; fat: 95 percent.

Berry Nut Butter

Brighten the flavor of your fat bombs with this luscious and fruity Berry Nut Butter.

3/4 cup (110 g/3.9 oz) blanched almonds

2/3 cup (90 g/3.2 oz) macadamia nuts

1/2 cup (125 g/4.4 oz) coconut butter

1/2 cup (110 g/3.9 oz) coconut oil

3/4 cup (60 g/2.1 oz) freeze-dried berry powder (raspberry, strawberry, blackberry, or blueberry) or equivalent weight of whole freeze-dried berries

Few drops liquid stevia, to taste (optional)

1. In a food processor, combine the almonds, macadamia nuts, and coconut butter. Add the stevia (if using), and process until smooth. The exact amount of time depends on your processor.

2. Add the coconut oil and berry powder. Pulse again until combined. Spoon the butter into a glass container. Seal and store for 1 week at room temperature or refrigerate for up to 3 months. Note that the butter will become liquid at room temperature.

YIELD: about 2 cups (500 g/8.8 oz)

....

NUTRITIONAL FACTS

Per serving (2 tablespoons [1.1 ounce, or 32 g]): total carbs: 6.4 g; fiber: 3.6 g; net carbs: 2.7 g; protein: 2.8 g; fat: 19.7 g; energy: 197 kcal.

Macronutrient ratio: calories from carbs: 5 percent; protein: 6 percent; fat: 89 percent.

Create your own nut butter creations by replacing the berry powder with these alternatives: 1/4 cup (25 g/0.9 oz) of beetroot powder, 1 to 2 tablespoons (8 to 16 g/ 0.3 to 0.6 oz) of pumpkin spice mix, or 1 to 2 teaspoons of turmeric.

Spiced Maple and Pecan Butter

The combination of maple, pecan, and cinnamon smacks of a cool, crisp fall morning, and this sugar-free nut butter captures those rich, spicy flavors to enjoy any time.

3 cups (300 g/10.6 oz) pecans

1 to 2 teaspoons natural maple extract

1/2 teaspoon ground cinnamon

1 teaspoon sugar-free vanilla extract or 1/2 teaspoon vanilla powder

Pinch salt

In a food processor, combine the pecans, maple extract, cinnamon, vanilla, and salt. Process until smooth. The exact amount of time depends on your processor. Spoon the butter into a glass container. Seal and store at room temperature for up to 1 week or refrigerate for up to 3 months.

YIELD: about 1 cups (310 g/10.9 oz)

....

NUTRITIONAL FACTS

Per serving (2 tablespoons [1.1 ounce, or 32g]): total carbs: 4.6 g; fiber: 3.1 g; net carbs: 1.4 g; protein: 2.9 g; fat: 22.3 g; energy: 216 kcal.

Macronutrient ratio: calories from carbs: 3 percent; protein: 5 percent; fat: 92 percent.

▶ For fat bomb-friendly food extracts, use unsweetened food extracts that are free from propylene glycol and any added sugar. Other common ingredients found in food extracts include water, natural oils, alcohol, and glycerin. Avoid using alcohol if your primary aim is to lose weight, but small amounts in food extracts won't do any harm. Another ingredient that turns up is glycerin, which is a liquid byproduct of making soap. It belongs to a special category of carbohydrates called polyols. Glycerin has a minimal effect on blood sugar levels and can be used in small quantities. Certain food extracts can also be swapped for a few drops of essential oils, such as orange, lemon, and mint.

Chocolate Chip Cookie Butter

There's no need to say goodbye to cookies—or chocolate—when you're eating low carb. This decadent butter is the proof, and it's sure to become an absolute favorite!

FOR COOKIES:

1½ cups (150 g/5.3 oz) almond flour

⅓ cup (50 g/1.8 oz) erythritol or Swerve

½ teaspoon baking soda mixed with 1 teaspoon cream of tartar, or 1 teaspoon gluten-free baking powder

Pinch salt

1 teaspoon sugar-free vanilla extract or ½ teaspoon vanilla powder

1 teaspoon freshly grated lemon zest

2 large egg yolks

2 tablespoons (30 g/1.1 oz) butter or ghee, at room temperature

FOR COOKIE BUTTER:

Crushed cookies (recipe follows)

½ cup (112 g/4 oz) unsalted butter or ghee or coconut oil, at room temperature

½ cup (90 g/3.2 oz) dark chocolate chips, 85 percent cacao solids or more, or make your own (see Homemade Dark Chocolate [page 32])

Few drops liquid stevia, to taste (optional)

1. Preheat the oven to 300°F (150°C, or gas mark 2).

2. To make the cookies: In a mixing bowl, combine the almond flour, erythritol, baking soda and cream of tartar, and salt. Mix well to combine. Add the vanilla, lemon zest, egg yolks, and butter. Mix together well with your hands.

3. Place the dough on a sheet of parchment paper. Top with another sheet of parchment and roll out to create a large cookie about ¼ inch (6.5 mm) thick. Transfer to a baking sheet and it in the preheated oven. Bake for 12 to 15 minutes, or until lightly browned and crispy. Remove from the oven and cool to room temperature. When cool, break into smaller pieces.

4. To make the cookie butter: In a food processor, pulse together the cookie pieces and butter until smooth. Add the chocolate chips. For a sweeter taste, add the stevia (if using). Pulse quickly to combine. Transfer to a sealed container and refrigerate for up to 1 week.

YIELD: about 1 cups (470 g/16.6 oz)

NUTRITIONAL FACTS

Per serving (2 tablespoons [1.1 ounce, or 32 g]): total carbs: 3.9 g; fiber: 1.5 g; net carbs: 2.4 g; protein: 3.3 g; fat: 16.6 g; energy: 170 kcal.

Macronutrient ratio: calories from carbs: 6 percent; protein: 8 percent; fat: 87 percent.

▶ Instead of vanilla extract and lemon, try cinnamon or pumpkin spice mix and freshly grated orange zest.

Pistachio-Coconut Butter

Pistachio nuts are like potato chips—it's impossible to eat just one. Get your fix with this creamy nut butter that's packed with pistachios, macadamia nuts, and coconut.

1 cup (120 g/4.2 oz) pistachio nuts

1 cup (75 g/2.6 oz) shredded unsweetened coconut

1 cup (130 g/4.7 oz) macadamia nuts

1 teaspoon sugar-free vanilla extract or ½ teaspoon vanilla powder

Pinch salt

In a food processor, combine the pistachios, coconut, macadamia nuts, vanilla, and salt. Pulse until smooth. The exact amount of time depends on your processor. Spoon the butter into a glass container. Seal and store at room temperature for up to 1 week or refrigerate for up to 3 months.

YIELD: about 1⅓ cups (330 g/11.6 oz)

....
NUTRITIONAL FACTS

Per serving (2 tablespoons [1.1 ounce, or 32 g]): total carbs: 6.7 g; fiber: 3.5 g; net carbs: 3.2 g; protein: 4.8 g; fat: 15.8 g; energy: 182 kcal.

Macronutrient ratio: calories from carbs: 7 percent; protein: 11 percent; fat: 82 percent.

▶ Intensify the flavor of this butter by using toasted pistachios, macadamias, and coconut. Preheat the oven to 350°F (175°C, or gas mark 4). Spread the pistachios, macadamias, and coconut on a baking sheet. Place it in the preheated oven and toast for 5 to 8 minutes, or until the coconut is lightly golden. Stir once or twice to prevent burning. The pistachios will turn light brown, instead of green, and the flavor will be more intense.

Pumpkin Sun Butter

Can't eat nuts? Never fear: you can still make fat bombs with this spiced, nut-free seed butter.

1½ cups (210 g/7.4 oz) sunflower seeds

½ cup (65 g/2.3 oz) pumpkin seeds

2 teaspoons ground cinnamon

Pinch salt

In a food processor, combine the sunflower seeds, pumpkin seeds, cinnamon, and salt. Pulse until smooth. The exact amount of time depends on your processor. Spoon the butter into a glass container. Seal and store at room temperature for up to 1 week, or refrigerate for up to 3 months.

YIELD: about 1 cups (280 g/9.9 oz)

....

NUTRITIONAL FACTS

Per serving (2 tablespoons [1.1 ounce, or 32 g]): total carbs: 6.1 g; fiber: 2.8 g; net carbs: 3.3 g; protein: 7.3 g; fat: 16 g; energy: 183 kcal.

Macronutrient ratio: calories from carbs: 7 percent; protein: 16 percent; fat: 77 percent.

Almond Bliss Butter

This treat will remind you of those fun-size candy bars you got in your Halloween goodie bag. If you adored those chocolate-coated, almond-studded delights, you'll feel like a kid again when you try this rich, delicious nut butter.

2 cups (150 g/5.3 oz) unsweetened shredded coconut

1/2 cup (75 g/2.6 oz) almonds

2.5 ounces (70 g) dark chocolate, 85 percent cacao solids or more

2.5 ounces (70 g) cacao butter

1/4 cup (40 g/1.4 oz) erythritol or Swerve

Few drops liquid stevia, to taste (optional)

1. Preheat the oven to 350°F (175°C, or gas mark 4). Spread the coconut and almonds on a baking sheet. Place it in the preheated oven and roast for 5 to 8 minutes, or until the coconut is lightly golden. Stir once or twice to prevent burning. Remove from the oven and set aside for a few minutes to cool.

2. In a food processor, combine the coconut, almonds, dark chocolate, cacao butter, and erythritol. Pulse until smooth. The exact amount of time depends on your processor. Add the stevia (if using), and pulse again. Spoon the butter into a glass container. Seal and store at room temperature for up to 1 week, or refrigerate for up to 3 months.

YIELD: about 1 ⅔ cups (405 g/14.3 oz)

....

NUTRITIONAL FACTS

Per serving (2 tablespoons [1.1 ounce, or 32 g]): total carbs: 5.9 g; fiber: 3.2 g; net carbs: 2.8 g; protein: 4.4 g; fat: 11.8 g; energy: 147 kcal.

Macronutrient ratio: calories from carbs: 8 percent; protein: 12 percent; fat: 80 percent.

Homemade Dark Chocolate Three Ways

Make healthy, sugar-free chocolate in a few simple steps.

FOR DARK CHOCOLATE USING UNSWEETENED CHOCOLATE (makes 8 ounces, or 225 g):

3 ounces (85 g) unsweetened chocolate

3 ounces (85 g) cacao butter

⅓ cup (50 g/1.8 oz) erythritol or Swerve, powdered

1 teaspoon sugar-free vanilla extract or ½ teaspoon vanilla powder

Pinch salt

Few drops liquid stevia, to taste (optional)

FOR DARK CHOCOLATE USING CACAO POWDER (makes 7.5 ounces, or 210 g):

4 ounces (112 g) cacao butter

½ cup (40 g/1.4 oz) unsweetened cacao powder

⅓ cup (50 g/1.8 oz) erythritol or Swerve, powdered

1 teaspoon sugar-free vanilla extract or ½ teaspoon vanilla powder

Pinch salt

Few drops liquid stevia, to taste (optional)

FOR DARK CHOCOLATE USING COCONUT OIL (makes 6.8 ounces, or 195 g):

½ cup (110 g/3.9 oz) coconut oil

½ cup (40 g/1.5 oz) unsweetened cacao powder

¼ cup (40 g/1.4 oz) erythritol or Swerve, powdered

1 teaspoon sugar-free vanilla extract or ½ teaspoon vanilla powder

Pinch salt

Few drops liquid stevia, to taste (optional)

1. *To make dark chocolate using unsweetened chocolate:* Melt the unsweetened chocolate and cacao butter in a double boiler, or heat-proof bowl placed over a small saucepan filled with 1 cup (235 ml) of water, over medium heat. Remove from the heat and set aside. Stir in the erythritol, vanilla, and salt. If you want a sweeter taste, add the stevia. Pour the chocolate into candy or chocolate molds or onto a parchment-lined baking sheet. Let it harden at room temperature, or in the refrigerator. Remove from the molds. Store at room temperature or refrigerate for up to 3 months.

2. *To make dark chocolate using cacao powder:* Melt the cacao butter in a double boiler, or heat-proof bowl placed over a small saucepan filled with 1 cup (235 ml) of water, over medium heat. Remove from the heat and set aside. Stir in the cacao powder, erythritol, vanilla, and salt. If you want a

sweeter taste, add the stevia. Pour into candy or chocolate molds and harden at room temperature or in the refrigerator. Once hardened, remove from the molds and keep in an airtight container. Store at room temperature or refrigerate for up to 3 months.

3. *To make dark chocolate using coconut oil:* Melt the coconut oil in a double boiler, or heat-proof bowl placed over a small saucepan filled with 1 cup (235 ml) of water, over medium heat. Once melted, add the cacao powder, erythritol, vanilla, and salt. If you want a sweeter taste, add the stevia. Pour into candy or chocolate molds and harden in the refrigerator. Once hardened, remove from the molds and store in an airtight container. Always store in the refrigerator: coconut oil melts at room temperature. Refrigerate for up to 3 months or freeze for up to 6 months.

YIELD: dark chocolate using unsweetened chocolate: 8 ounces, or 225

YIELD: dark chocolate using cacao powder: 7.5 ounces, or 213 g

YIELD: dark chocolate using coconut oil: 6.8 ounces, or 195 g

NUTRITIONAL FACTS

Per serving of each type (1 ounce, or 28 g): total carbs: 3 g/3.5 g/3.7 g; fiber: 1.5 g/1.8 g/1.9 g; net carbs: 1.5 g/1.7 g/1.8 g; protein: 1.5 g/1.1 g/1.1 g; fat: 16.2 g/15.9 g/16.4 g; energy: 164 kcal/150 kcal/151 kcal.

Macronutrient ratio: calories from carbs: 6 percent/5 percent/5 percent; protein: 4 percent/3 percent/3 percent; fat: 92 percent/93 percent/93 percent.

Homemade White Chocolate

Packed with healthy fats and made from real food ingredients (no additives here!), this Homemade White Chocolate is sugar-free and infused with fragrant vanilla.

6 ounces (170 g) cacao butter

1 cup (120 g/4.2 oz) coconut milk powder

⅓ cup (50 g/1.8 oz) erythritol or Swerve, powdered

2 teaspoons sugar-free vanilla extract or 1 teaspoon vanilla powder

Pinch salt

Few drops liquid stevia, to taste (optional)

Melt the cacao butter in a double boiler, or heat-proof bowl placed over a small saucepan filled with 1 cup (235 ml) of water, over medium heat. Remove from the heat and set aside. Add the coconut milk powder, and lucuma powder (if using; see Note), erythritol, vanilla, and salt. If you want a sweeter taste, add the stevia. Pour the mixture into a food processor. Pulse for 30 to 60 seconds, or until smooth. Pour into candy or chocolate molds and let the chocolate harden in the refrigerator. Once solid, remove from the molds. Store at room temperature or refrigerate for up to 3 months.

YIELD: about 12 ounces, or 340 g

....

NUTRITIONAL FACTS

Per serving (1 ounce, or 28 g): total carbs: 2.7 g; fiber: 0.1 g; net carbs: 2.6 g; protein: 0.7 g; fat: 19.8 g; energy: 191 kcal.

Macronutrient ratio: calories from carbs: 5 percent; protein: 1 percent; fat: 93 percent.

▶ For an extra nutritional boost, swap ½ cup (60 g/0.9 oz) of coconut milk powder with ½ cup (40 g/1.4 oz) of lucuma powder: What is lucuma powder? Lucuma, a sub-tropical fruit, is an anti-inflammatory superfood also known as "Gold of the Incas." It's high in carotene, iron, vitamin B3, and fiber, and has a light orange color. The powder made from this fruit adds natural sweetness to the chocolate, and makes it creamier. Keep in mind that lucuma powder has more than twice as many carbs as coconut milk powder, so stick to the suggested amounts. Using lucuma powder in this recipe will result in 4.3 grams of net carbs Per serving.

2

SCHOOL AND WORK SNACKS:
Nourishing Noshes to
Fuel Your Day

Study after study has shown that consuming high-carbohydrate, high-glycemic foods spikes insulin, leading to a postmeal crash in both energy and focus. Ever wonder why you want to take a nap about an hour after a slice of pizza?

Fortunately, science is homing in on how our food can help us focus.

You may have heard about the importance of protein in our diet, but only recently have we come to understand what a huge role high-protein foods play in our mental health. Studies show that protein improves concentration levels. It elevates dopamine, which regulates happiness, and neurotransmitters that help brain cells "talk" with each other and function properly. Research also suggests that high-protein diets may reduce symptoms of ADHD and improve behavior and attention.

By consuming snacks that include beneficial fatty acids such as omega-3s, which are crucial to a well-functioning brain, concentration can be improved. Because the body can't produce omega 3-s, we need to get them from our diet—walnuts and flaxseeds are great options. One particular type of omega-3 is DHA, which has been shown in some studies to have a direct impact on ADHD and concentration levels.

Likewise, it is hard to stay focused at work or school if your tummy is rumbling. Snacks with a healthy amount of fiber can help you stay satiated for extended periods. Fiber comes in two forms: soluble and insoluble. While insoluble fiber passes through the digestive system relatively untouched, soluble fiber, the kind found in nuts, flaxseeds, and psyllium husk, absorbs water in your stomach and gut, thereby helping you feel full longer.

This chapter contains recipes that are optimized for heightened concentration, a consistent level of energy, and staving off hunger to help you be the best you (and your children, if you have them) can be at work or school. Not just superhealthy, most of these snacks are also nut-free, which make them nice options in "peanut/nut-free" schools or workplaces.

Savory Baked Chicken Nuggets

Chicken nuggets are always a favorite with the kids, but you know you love them too! They are supertasty and an excellent source of protein, which keeps that concentration level up all day. Try making a double batch and store them in the freezer in an airtight bag or container.

1 pound (455 g) chicken breasts (about 3 large breasts), cut into bite-size pieces

¼ cup (55 g) grass-fed butter, melted

1 cup (100 g) almond meal or cashew flour

3 tablespoons (24 g) sesame seeds

1 tablespoon (7 g) paprika

2 teaspoons onion powder

1½ teaspoons salt

1 teaspoon garlic powder

¼ teaspoon cayenne pepper

1. Preheat the oven to 400°F (200°C, or gas mark 6). Place a wire rack in a baking sheet or baking dish. (If you don't have a wire rack, line the baking sheet with parchment paper.)

2. Place the melted butter in a small bowl. In a separate small bowl, mix together the almond meal, sesame seeds, paprika, onion powder, salt, garlic powder, and cayenne pepper.

3. Put five or so pieces of chicken in the bowl with butter and coat them well. Then put the chicken into the bowl with the spices and coat evenly. Set the chicken on the wire rack or parchment paper and repeat the process until all of your chicken is coated.

4. Bake for 10 minutes. Then turn the oven to broil, and bake another 4 or 5 minutes, until golden brown. You don't have to flip them (thanks goodness, because it's a pain!).

5. Nuggets store well in the fridge for 3 to 4 days or in the freezer for up to 6 months.

YIELD: about 24 nuggets

NUTRITIONAL FACTS

Per nugget: total carbs: 1.6 g; fiber: 0.8 g; net carbs: 0.8 g; protein: 5.6 g; fat: 5.5 g; calories: 76.

Macronutrient ratio: calories from carbs: 8 percent; protein: 29 percent; fat: 63 percent.

Sun-Dried Tomato Chicken Sliders

This flavorful slider is a fun alternative to a traditional chicken burger. And because it's all protein, it's a great snack to keep your concentration going strong.

1 pound (455 g) ground chicken

½ of a small onion, finely chopped

2 tablespoons (14 g) sundried tomatoes packed in oil, chopped

2 tablespoons (5 g) fresh basil, chopped

2 cloves of garlic, pressed

2 teaspoons salt

1 teaspoon ground black pepper

2 tablespoons (27 g) coconut oil

1. In a medium bowl, combine the chicken, onion, sundried tomatoes, basil, garlic, salt, and pepper until well combined. To form sliders, take a spoonful of the mixture and pat together a patty that is 2 to 3 inches (5 to 7.5 cm) in diameter.

2. Heat a large pan over medium-high and add the coconut oil. Carefully place patties in the pan, as many as you can without touching. Once the patties start to brown, carefully turn them, and cook for a few more minutes so they can brown. Then turn the heat down to low and cook for about 7 more minutes, or until no longer pink in the middle. Snack on them as is, or turn them into a meal by using them to top a salad.

YIELD: about 15 sliders

....

NUTRITIONAL FACTS

Per slider: total carbs: 0.7 g; fiber: 0.1 g; net carbs: 0.5 g; protein: 5 g; fat: 4 g; calories: 63.

Macronutrient ratio: calories from carbs: 4 percent; protein: 34 percent; fat: 62 percent.

Chicken Maple Sausage Meatballs

Studies show that protein helps with concentration, and these easy-to-eat, kid- and adult-friendly mini meatballs are an easy way to get more protein in our bodies. To make these nut-free, substitute 1 tablespoon (7 g) coconut flour for the almond meal.

1 pound (455 g) hormone-free ground chicken

1 egg

2 tablespoons (12 g) almond meal

1 tablespoon (20 g) maple syrup

1 teaspoon salt

1 teaspoon garlic powder

1 teaspoon paprika

1 teaspoon Dijon mustard

1/2 teaspoon dried rosemary

1/2 teaspoon dried thyme

1. Preheat the oven to 400°F (200°C, or gas mark 6). Line a baking sheet with parchment paper.

2. In a medium bowl, combine the chicken, egg, almond meal, maple syrup, salt, garlic powder, paprika, mustard, rosemary, and thyme. With your hands, make golf ball–size balls out of the mixture and lay on the prepared baking sheet. Bake for 18 to 20 minutes, until cooked through.

YIELD: about 15 meatballs

....

NUTRITIONAL FACTS

Per meatball: total carbs: 1.6 g; fiber: 0.2 g; net carbs: 1.4 g; protein: 6 g; fat: 3.2 g; calories: 59.

Macronutrient ratio: calories from carbs: 11 percent; protein: 40 percent; fat: 49 percent.

Buffalo Chicken Wings

Ready for a little spice? Traditional buffalo wings are delicious, but too often they are fried in unhealthy oils and coated with gluten. This wonderful recipe is a Paleo twist on a favorite party snack.

2¾ pounds (1 kg) raw chicken wings

½ cup (64 g) arrowroot powder

1 teaspoon salt

½ teaspoon garlic powder

½ teaspoon cayenne pepper (optional)

½ cup (112 g) grass-fed butter

½ cup gluten-free hot sauce (such as Texas Pete's)

1. Set the wings on a few paper towels and pat dry. In a resealable plastic freezer bag, combine the arrowroot, salt, garlic powder, and cayenne (if using). Add the wings to the bag, and shake until well coated. Set the wings on a wire rack on a baking sheet, and place in the fridge for 1 hour to help the wings absorb the spices and prevent sogginess.

2. Preheat the oven to 400°F (200°C, or gas mark 6).

3. After the hour of refrigeration, bake the wings for 20 minutes. Turn the wings over and bake for another 20 minutes. While the wings bake, in a small saucepan, melt the butter and stir in the hot sauce until well combined. Set aside. As it sits, it will thicken up, which will add more flavor to the wings.

4. Take the wings out of the oven and brush them with the sauce. Return to the oven and bake for an additional 10 minutes. Broil them for the last minute or two to get them crispy.

YIELD: about 2 dozen wings

....

NUTRITIONAL FACTS

Per wing: total carbs: 3.6 g; fiber: 0.1 g; net carbs: 3.5 g; protein: 5 g; fat: 7.5 g; calories: 103.

Macronutrient ratio: calories from carbs: 14 percent; protein: 20 percent; fat: 66 percent.

Italian Meatballs

Not only does grass-fed meat contain lots of iron, but it also has many powerful nutrients that help build strong bones and a strong immune system. It also provides a good source of steady energy and concentration, and on top of that, it burns belly fat from its abundant CLA (conjugated linoleic acid), a fatty acid. Talk about a perfect snack. These absolutely delicious meatballs don't need any messy tomato sauce, which makes them perfect for packing.

1 pound (455 g) grass-fed ground beef

1/2 pound (225 g) ground Italian sausage (removed from casing if needed)

1/2 of a small onion, finely chopped or grated

2 eggs

2 cloves of garlic, minced

1/4 cup (28 g) almond meal or flour

3 tablespoons (12 g) fresh parsley, finely chopped

1 1/2 teaspoons salt

1 teaspoon ground black pepper

1 teaspoon dried basil

1 teaspoon dried oregano

1. Preheat the oven to 350°F (180°C, or gas mark 4).

2. In a medium bowl, mix together the beef, sausage, onion, eggs, garlic, almond meal, parsley, salt, pepper, basil, and oregano by hand. Form the meatballs about 3 inches (7.5 cm) in diameter.

3. Add the meatballs to a large cast iron skillet (or other ovenproof skillet) over medium-high heat. Cook until they are browned on all sides. Then place the skillet in the oven (or transfer the meatballs to a baking sheet) and bake for an additional 10 minutes.

YIELD: about 15 meatballs

....

NUTRITIONAL FACTS

Per meatball: total carbs: 1.6 g; fiber: 0.4 g; net carbs: 1.3 g; protein: 10.1 g; fat: 9.6 g; calories: 134.

Macronutrient ratio: calories from carbs: 5 percent; protein: 30 percent; fat: 65 percent.

Homemade Beef Jerky

Beef jerky is a great and easy way to get a lot of protein. Unfortunately, most jerky available in grocery stores are made with meat containing hormones and antibiotics. In addition, they are typically full of sugar, gluten/wheat, and unhealthy preservatives. Instead, try this healthy, incredibly easy alternative. It only requires a little prep work, and it's so worth it!

2½ pounds (1.1 kg) grass-fed London broil (flank steak or any lean meat)

1 cup (235 ml) gluten-free tamari soy sauce or coconut aminos

1 tablespoon (20 g) dark raw honey

2 teaspoons onion powder

1 teaspoon garlic powder

1 teaspoon salt

Place meat in the freezer for 1 to 2 hours to make it easier to slice. Remove from freezer and trim off any visible fat. Then slice it against the grain into thin strips (about ¼ inch [6.5 mm] thick).

1. In a plastic freezer bag, combine the soy sauce, honey, onion powder, garlic powder, and salt. Add the meat and marinate for at least 4 hours, preferably overnight.

2. Preheat the oven to 170°F (76°C), if you aren't using a dehydrator. On a parchment-lined baking sheet, lay the meat out flat, but make sure none of it is touching or overlapping.

3. Cook for 4 to 6 hours (it will depend on thickness), until desired texture. Flip the meat once or twice while cooking. If using a dehydrator, allow it to dehydrate for 4 to 5 hours.

4. Store the jerky in the fridge or freezer, but it is fine to keep at room temperature for a couple of days.

YIELD: 20 to 25 pieces

....

NUTRITIONAL FACTS

Per piece (2 oz, or 62 g): total carbs: 0.6 g; fiber: 0.1 g; net carbs: 0.5 g; protein: 12.5 g; fat: 3.7 g; calories: 89.

Macronutrient ratio: calories from carbs: 3 percent; protein: 58 percent; fat: 39 percent.

Bacon Cauliflower Soup

Because cauliflower has choline, a B vitamin that is essential for your brain's neurotransmitters and can help with focus, this soup is a great snack during the school or work day.

6 to 8 slices nitrate-free bacon

1 small yellow onion, roughly chopped

2 cloves of garlic

1 large or 2 small heads of cauliflower, roughly chopped

About 1 quart (946 ml) lower-sodium chicken broth

1 tablespoon (18 g) salt

1 teaspoon ground black pepper

About 2/3 cup (160 ml) unsweetened canned light coconut milk

1. Cut the bacon into pieces (about four or five pieces per slice, but slice it all together to save time). Put it in a large pot and cook over medium-high heat until it starts to get crispy. Add the onion and garlic, and sauté for a couple of minutes until they start to brown. Continuously stir.

2. Add the cauliflower, chicken broth (fill it so it covers the cauliflower by about 2 inches, or 5 cm), salt, and pepper to the pot. Bring to a boil, then turn the heat down to low and cover with the lid. Cook until the cauliflower starts to become soft, about 10 minutes.

3. Stir in the coconut milk, then carefully transfer to a high-speed blender (in batches, if necessary). You can also use an immersion blender, which is easier and less messy, but you won't get quite as creamy and fluffy a result. Blend on high for 60 to 90 seconds, until creamy and very smooth. Return to the pot and heat through.

4. Enjoy with some spicy sausage, chives, more bacon, and/or cheese or whatever you prefer. Or, just enjoy it as is. It's good any way! When storing soup in a plastic container, make sure the soup is cool and the container is BPA-free.

YIELD: 2½ quarts (2.5 L)

NUTRITIONAL FACTS

Per serving (8 oz, or 227 g): total carbs: 5.8 g; fiber: 1.9 g; net carbs: 3.9 g; protein: 4.9 g; fat: 3.7 g; calories: 73

Macronutrient ratio: calories from carbs: 31 percent; protein: 26 percent; fat: 44 percent.

Cauliflower Pizza Bites

This gluten-free pizza crust can be turned into mini, easy-to-eat pizzas. It just so happens that this is the healthiest pizza crust around. With six different types of B vitamins for energy, lots of vitamin C, and a load of antioxidants, this is a super snack.

1 large head of cauliflower, cored and broken into large florets

1 egg

4 ounces (115 g) soft goat cheese (Chevre)

1 tablespoon (3 g) dried oregano

1 teaspoon salt

Optional toppings:

Tomato or pizza sauce

Parmesan or mozzarella cheese

Olives, pepperoni, etc.

1. Preheat the oven to 400°F (200°C, or gas mark 6). Grease a 12-cup mini-muffin pan.

2. In a food processor, chop the cauliflower until it is a rice-like consistency. Bring a pot of water to a boil. Add the cauliflower and cook it for 6 to 8 minutes, until soft. Strain and rinse with cold water. Lay out a clean kitchen towel. Pour the "rice" onto the towel, wrap the towel around the "rice," and twist it and squeeze out as much water as you can.

3. In a medium bowl, beat the egg and add the goat cheese, oregano, and salt. Add the cauliflower "rice" and blend it all together with your hands. It's messy, but it works best this way.

4. Evenly spoon mixture into the muffin cups, filling them close to the top. Press down the dough evenly and firmly to ensure it sticks together. Bake for 15 to 18 minutes, or until the tops start to turn a light brown. Remove from the oven and let cool in the pan for at least 10 minutes.

5. Dip in tomato sauce or add whatever toppings you desire.

YIELD: 12 pizza bites

NUTRITIONAL FACTS

Per bite: total carbs: 3.7 g; fiber: 1.5 g; net carbs: 2.2 g; protein: 3.6 g; fat: 2.7 g; calories: 50.

Macronutrient ratio: calories from carbs: 28 percent; protein: 27 percent; fat: 45 percent.

Herbed Cheese Fat Bombs

Reach for one of these cheesy fat bombs the next time you're craving a snack. They're infused with garlic and fresh herbs and coated in Parmesan cheese, and they're incredibly satisfying.

3.5 ounces (100 g) full-fat cream cheese, at room temperature

¼ cup (56 g/2 oz) unsalted butter, at room temperature

4 pieces (12 g /0.4 oz) sun-dried tomatoes, drained and chopped

4 (12 g/0.4 oz) pitted olives, such as kalamatas, chopped

2 to 3 tablespoons (10 g/0.4 oz) chopped fresh herbs (such as basil, thyme, and oregano), or 2 teaspoons dried herbs

2 cloves of garlic, crushed

Salt and pepper, to taste

5 tablespoons (25 g /0.9 oz) grated Parmesan cheese

1. In a bowl, mash together the cream cheese and butter, or process in a food processor until smooth.

2. Add the sun-dried tomatoes, olives, herbs, and garlic. Season with salt and pepper. Mix well to combine. Refrigerate for 20 to 30 minutes, or until set.

3. Using a large spoon or an ice cream scoop, divide the mixture into five balls. Roll each ball in the Parmesan cheese. Enjoy immediately or refrigerate in an airtight container for up to 1 week.

YIELD: 5 servings

NUTRITIONAL FACTS

Per serving: total carbs: 2 g; fiber: 0.3 g; net carbs: 1.7 g; protein: 3.7 g; fat: 17.1 g; energy: 164 kcal.

Macronutrient ratio: calories from carbs: 4 percent; protein: 8 percent; fat: 88 percent.

Salmon Pâté Fat Bombs

Smoked salmon and cream cheese—partners in crime—are at their best when dressed up with lemon and dill. This simple recipe shows you how to transform that classic combination into fabulous, keto-friendly fat bombs.

3.5 ounces (100 g) full-fat cream cheese, at room temperature

1/3 cup (75 g /2.7 oz) unsalted butter or ghee, at room temperature

1 small package (50 g /1.8 oz) smoked salmon

1 tablespoon (15 ml/0.5 fl oz) fresh lemon juice

2 tablespoons (8 g/0.3 oz) chopped fresh dill, plus additional for garnishing

Salt and pepper, to taste

Crispy lettuce leaves, for serving (optional)

1. In a food processor, combine the cream cheese, butter, smoked salmon, lemon juice, and dill. Pulse until smooth.

2. Line a baking sheet with parchment paper. Spoon about 2 tablespoons (40 g/1.4 oz) of the mixture per portion onto the prepared sheet. Garnish each with more dill. Refrigerate for 20 to 30 minutes, or until set. Alternatively, transfer the mixture to an airtight container and refrigerate. When ready to serve, spoon out 2 tablespoons (40 g/1.4 oz) Per serving and serve on top of lettuce leaves. Keep refrigerated in an airtight container for up to 1 week.

YIELD: 6 servings

....

NUTRITIONAL FACTS

Per serving: total carbs: 0.8 g; fiber: 0.1 g; net carbs: 0.7 g; protein: 3.2 g; fat: 15.7 g; energy: 147 kcal

Macronutrient ratio: calories from carbs: 2 percent; protein: 8 percent; fat: 90 percent.

Anchovy Fat Bombs

Anchovies, though not for everyone, are packed with healthy fats. Try them in this easy-to-prepare tapenade, where their assertiveness is balanced by other strong flavors such as garlic, parsley, and cheese.

3.5 ounces (100 g) full-fat cream cheese, at room temperature

¼ cup (56 g/2 oz) unsalted butter, at room temperature

1 ounce (28 g) canned anchovies, drained

1 clove of garlic, crushed

1 tablespoon (3 g/0.1 oz) chopped fresh parsley

¼ cup (28 g/1 oz) shredded Cheddar cheese

⅓ cup (30 g/1.1 oz) flaked almonds

Cucumber slices, for serving (optional)

In a food processor, combine the cream cheese, butter, anchovies, garlic, and parsley. Pulse until smooth. Transfer to a bowl and add the Cheddar cheese and almonds and mix with a spoon. Refrigerate for 20 to 30 minutes, or until set. Enjoy as a dip with sliced cucumber, or keep refrigerated in an airtight container for up to 1 week.

YIELD: 6 servings

NUTRITIONAL FACTS

Per serving: total carbs: 1.8 g; fiber: 0.7 g; net carbs: 1.1 g; protein: 5.1 g; fat: 17.2 g; energy: 170 kcal.

Macronutrient ratio: calories from carbs: 3 percent; protein: 11 percent.

Chorizo and Avocado Fat Bombs

Load crispy bits of chorizo and diced hardboiled eggs into avocado halves for filling fat bombs that double as a quick low-carb lunch or brunch.

3.5 ounces (100 g) Spanish chorizo sausage, diced

2 large hardboiled eggs, cooled, peeled, and diced

¼ cup (56 g /2 oz) unsalted butter, at room temperature

2 tablespoons (30 g/1.1 oz) mayonnaise, preferably homemade

1 tablespoon (15 ml/0.5 fl oz) freshly squeezed lemon juice

2 tablespoons (8 g/0.3 oz) chopped fresh chives

Salt and cayenne pepper, to taste

4 large (400 g /14.1 oz) avocado halves, pitted

1. In a hot pan, fry the chorizo for a few minutes until crispy. Remove from the heat and set aside.

2. In a mixing bowl, combine the eggs, chorizo (reserving a small amount for topping), and the butter. Mash together with a fork. Add the mayonnaise, lemon juice, and chives. Season with salt and cayenne pepper. Mix with a fork to combine. Refrigerate for 20 to 30 minutes, or until set.

3. Just before serving, top each avocado half with one-quarter of the egg and chorizo mixture. Sprinkle with the reserved chorizo and enjoy immediately. Keep the egg and chorizo mixture refrigerated in an airtight container for up to 5 days.

YIELD: 4 servings

....

NUTRITIONAL FACTS

Per serving (1 stuffed avocado half): total carbs: 9.5 g; fiber: 6.8 g; net carbs: 2.7 g; protein: 11.4 g; fat: 38.9 g; energy: 419 kcal.

Macronutrient ratio: calories from carbs: 3 percent; protein: 11 percent; fat: 86 percent.

Bacon & Egg Maple Muffins

With a sweet hint of maple and some salty bacon, this delectable snack is superfilling and satisfying. As it's made with an abundance of eggs, considered "brain food" by David Perlmutter, M.D., in his bestselling book Grain Brain, *this muffin clearly is an ideal snack.*

8 to 10 slices nitrate-free bacon

7 eggs, room temperature

1/4 cup (55 g) grass-fed butter, melted

2 tablespoons (40 g) maple syrup

1/2 cup (56 g) coconut flour

1/2 teaspoon salt

1/4 teaspoon baking soda

1/4 cup (60 ml) unsweetened canned coconut milk (stirred first)

1. Preheat the oven to 400°F (200°C, or gas mark 6). Place the bacon on a foil-lined baking sheet and bake for 8 to 10 minutes on each side. You want it to get really brown and crispy!

2. While the bacon bakes, in a medium bowl, mix together the eggs, butter, coconut milk, and maple syrup. In a small bowl, mix together the coconut flour, salt, and baking soda. Add to the egg mixture and stir well. Make sure you get all of the clumps out from the coconut flour.

3. When the bacon is done, place it on a paper towel to cool off a bit and then crumble it into the batter.

4. Reduce the heat to 350°F (180°C, or gas mark 4). Line a 12-cup muffin pan with silicone or paper muffin liners, or grease the cups. Fill the cups about two-thirds full. Bake for 20 minutes, or until a toothpick inserted in the middle of a muffin comes out clean.

5. These freeze well. Just pull one out the night before and place it in the fridge so it will be ready to go to school/work the next day. They're best when reheated but also yummy when eaten cool or at room temperature.

YIELD: 12 muffins

....
NUTRITIONAL FACTS

Per muffin: total carbs: 5.2 g; fiber: 1.7 g; net carbs: 3.5 g; protein: 6.4 g; fat: 10 g; calories: 139.

Macronutrient ratio: calories from carbs: 15 percent; protein: 19 percent; fat: 66 percent.

Pumpkin Chocolate Chip Muffins

This fall snack tastes amazing, but is also superhealthy. These muffins have lots of fiber from the coconut flour and pumpkin purée, tons of protein from the eggs, antioxidants from the dark chocolate, and good healthy brain fat from the coconut oil to boot.

3/4 cup (84 g) coconut flour

3/4 cup (144 g) coconut palm sugar

1 tablespoon (6.6 g) pumpkin pie spice

1 teaspoon ground cinnamon

3/4 teaspoon baking soda

1/2 teaspoon salt

9 eggs, room temperature

1/3 cup (82 g) pumpkin purée

2 tablespoons (40 g) maple syrup

1 teaspoon vanilla extract

2 tablespoons (28 ml) unsweetened canned coconut milk (stirred first)

1/3 cup (80 ml) coconut oil, melted

1 cup (175 g) dark chocolate chips

1. Preheat the oven to 350°F (180°C, or gas mark 4). Line eighteen cups of a muffin pan with silicone or paper muffin liners, or grease the cups.

2. In a medium bowl, mix together the coconut flour, coconut palm sugar, pumpkin pie spice, cinnamon, baking soda, and salt. In another bowl, whisk together the eggs, pumpkin purée, maple syrup, vanilla, and coconut milk. Add the wet ingredients to the dry and mix until well combined. Add the coconut oil and stir until smooth. Fold in the chocolate chips.

3. Pour the batter into the prepared muffin cups about two-thirds full. Bake for 23 to 25 minutes, or until a toothpick inserted in the middle of a muffin comes out clean, and eat while the chocolate is still melting!

4. These freeze well for up to 6 months.

YIELD: 18 muffins

....

NUTRITIONAL FACTS

Per muffin: total carbs: 21.2 g; fiber: 2.1 g; net carbs: 18.2 g; protein: 4.8 g; fat: 11.1 g; calories: 194.

Macronutrient ratio: calories from carbs: 42 percent; protein: 9 percent; fat: 49 percent.

Supersmart Bars

These taste like candy bars! But with the omega-3–rich walnuts, which can help with concentration, and the magnesium-packed cashews, which can help improve memory, this is the exact opposite of a candy bar. Further, the low-glycemic coconut nectar can help stabilize blood sugar levels, while the dark chocolate offers a little mental boost. This is an ideal snack for school or work!

1 cup (120 g) walnuts

1 cup (110 g) cashews

1 cup (80 g) unsweetened shredded coconut

2/3 cup (175 g) almond butter

1/3 cup (144 g) coconut oil

1/3 cup (115 g) coconut nectar

1 tablespoon (15 ml) vanilla extract

1/2 teaspoon salt

1/3 cup (58 g) dark chocolate chips

1. In a food processor, blend the walnuts, cashews, coconut, almond butter, coconut oil, coconut nectar, vanilla, and salt until the mixture starts to solidify. Then place the mixture into an 8 x 8 inch (20 x 20 cm) baking dish or pan and press firmly until flat and even. Place in the fridge for 30 to 60 minutes.

2. Set a small mixing bowl over a small pot of simmering water (be careful that the bowl does not touch the water). Put the chocolate chips in the bowl and stir until melted. Spread the chocolate over the bars and put back in the fridge until it hardens. Cut into 2 x 2 inch (5 x 5 cm) squares. You may want to use a metal spatula to get the squares out. The first one may be tricky to get out but the rest are easy. Store in the fridge.

YIELD: 12 bars

NUTRITIONAL FACTS

Per bar: total carbs: 14.2 g; fiber: 3.3 g; net carbs: 10.4 g; protein: 6.9 g; fat: 31.2 g; calories: 344.

Macronutrient ratio: calories from carbs: 16 percent; protein: 8 percent; fat: 76 percent.

3

AT-HOME SNACKS:
Skip the Chips for Delicious, Healthy Options

It is four in the afternoon. Dinner isn't for another couple of hours. You and your kids—if you have them—are hungry. You step to the pantry and stare into an unsatisfying abyss of prepackaged saltiness.

Like many people, you tear open a bag of chips or throw popcorn at the problem. The moment that bag rips open, you've lost. The endorphin rush of the first bite will lead to the second, then the third, and before you know it, there is no room left for a healthy dinner.

If any of this sounds familiar, this chapter will change your world.

There is a much healthier, tastier, and more satisfying approach to at-home snacks, and the recipes in this chapter are aimed at turning this traditionally nutritional void into something much more beneficial. All that is needed is less than 10 minutes of prep time and, potentially, a little marketing skill and resolve.

1. **Preparation:** If you are making and serving snacks at home, you have the advantage of an oven. Use that advantage to serve aromatic, warm snacks, which are more appetizing than something pulled from a box or bag. Conversely, on a warm summer day, retrieving a cool treat from the fridge will get everyone excited about snack time.

2. **Marketing:** Say this aloud: "It isn't a snack, it's an appetizer." After all, who doesn't love appetizers? That's what people eat at restaurants. Appetizers at home? What a delight. Likely, you and/or family will eat more kale chips (or whatever veggie) than if you had set them on their plates at dinnertime. This one is a win-win.

3. **Resolve:** Whether it is your family or yourself, change can be a struggle. If the norm is chips, and you prepare something new, don't relent. Let the new snack be the only snack.

A more likely test of your resolve will concern whether these healthy snacks, which are being aggressively devoured, are going to ruin everyone's appetite for dinner. With the veggie "appetizers," you don't have to worry about getting overly stuffed. Unlike traditional processed snacks, whole-food "appetizers" appropriately trigger satiation receptors in the brain so no one will overeat. Worst case, if they do, they will have filled up on nutritious vegetables. That is also a win-win.

Waldorf Salad Fat Bombs

There's only one thing to do when you've got pecans, cheese, and green apples lurking in your kitchen. Make these sugar-free, bite-size fat bombs!

3 ounces (85 g) full-fat cream cheese, at room temperature

2 tablespoons (28 g/1 oz) unsalted butter or ghee, at room temperature

1/2 cup (65 g/2.3 oz) crumbled blue cheese

1/2 of a small (60 g/2.1 oz) green apple, diced into 1/2 inch (1.5 cm) pieces

1/4 teaspoon garlic powder

1/4 teaspoon onion powder

2 tablespoons (5 g/0.2 oz) chopped fresh chives or spring onion

Salt and pepper, to taste

2/3 cup (70 g/2.5 oz) pecans or walnuts, roughly chopped

1. In a bowl, mash together the cream cheese and butter, or process in a food processor until smooth.

2. Add the crumbled blue cheese, apple, garlic powder, onion powder, and chives. Stir to combine. Season with salt and pepper. Refrigerate for 20 to 30 minutes, or until set.

3. Using a large spoon or an ice cream scoop, divide the mixture into six balls. Roll each ball in the pecans. Enjoy immediately or refrigerate in an airtight container for up to 1 week.

YIELD: 6 servings

NUTRITIONAL FACTS

Per serving: total carbs: 4 g; fiber: 1.5 g; net carbs: 2.5 g; protein: 4.5 g; fat: 19.3 g; energy: 193 kcal.

Macronutrient ratio: calories from carbs: 5 percent; protein: 9 percent; fat: 86 percent.

Kale Salad

Who knew kale could make such a delightfully mild and tasty salad? Because kale leaves don't get soggy and soak in flavor over time, this is a great recipe to make and store in your fridge for a delicious superfood snack any time. To make this salad nut-free, either omit the almonds or substitute roasted pepitas.

FOR SALAD:

1 bunch of Tuscan kale

1½ cups (132 g) brussels sprouts, grated or finely sliced (optional)

3 tablespoons (21 g) sliced almonds

3 tablespoons (23 g) dried cranberries

½ cup (50 g) grated Parmesan cheese

FOR DRESSING:

½ cup (120 ml) extra-virgin olive oil

3 tablespoons (45 ml) fresh lemon juice

1½ tablespoons (23 g) Dijon mustard

1 shallot, minced

2 small cloves of garlic, minced

1 teaspoon salt

Freshly ground black pepper, to taste

1. To make the salad: Remove the stems from the kale and roughly chop the leaves. You should have about 4 cups (220 g). Place in a large mixing bowl. Add the brussels sprouts, if using, along with the almonds, cranberries, and Parmesan.

2. To make the dressing: In a small bowl, mix together the olive oil, lemon juice, mustard, shallot, garlic, salt, and pepper. Pour the dressing over the kale mixture, and toss well. Let marinate in the fridge for at least 1 hour.

3. The salad lasts, covered, about 3 days in the fridge.

YIELD: 4 servings

....

NUTRITIONAL FACTS

Per serving (w/o brussels sprouts): total carbs: 10.1 g; fiber: 1.3 g; net carbs: 8.5 g; protein: 4.7 g; fat: 33.2 g; calories: 345.

Macronutrient ratio: calories from carbs: 11 percent; protein: 5 percent; fat: 83 percent.

Per serving (w/ brussels sprouts): total carbs: 13.1 g; fiber: 2.6 g; net carbs: 10.2 g; protein: 5.8 g; fat: 33.3 g; calories: 359.

Macronutrient ratio: calories from carbs: 14 percent; protein: 6 percent; fat: 80 percent.

Easy "Cheesy" Kale Chips

Kale chips can be a little tricky to make. The key is to tinker with your oven temperature until you can attain the right level of kale crispiness. Nutritional yeast is the perfect, nutrient-dense, and vitamin B–filled ingredient to make these chips have that yummy cheesy taste. No one will know they're superhealthy—or dairy-free!

1 bunch of kale

2 tablespoons (27 g) coconut oil, melted

¼ cup (28 g) cashew flour or crushed cashews

¼ cup (25 g) nutritional yeast

½ teaspoon salt

1. Preheat the oven to 300°F (150°C, or gas mark 2). Line a baking sheet with parchment paper.

2. Wash the kale and dry with paper towel. Cut the spine off each piece of kale and then cut the leaves in half. (Optional: Chop the kale into small pieces, if desired.) Place the leaves in a bowl with the coconut oil, and toss until the leaves are well coated. Set each piece of kale on the prepared baking sheet.

3. In a small bowl, mix together the cashew flour, nutritional yeast, and salt, and then sprinkle it over the kale to coat. Bake for 25 minutes.

4. Turn off the heat and let the chips sit in the oven, with the door closed, at least 30 minutes, until crisp. You might have to play with your oven to get just the right temp/time because everyone's oven is different.

5. You can bake them in the morning and let them sit in the oven for a couple of hours. By lunchtime, you will have optimally crunchy, warm kale chips waiting in the oven.

YIELD: about 8 servings

....

NUTRITIONAL FACTS

Per serving (1/2 oz, or 17K g): total carbs: 2.5 g; fiber: 0.8 g; net carbs: 1.7 g; protein: 1.8 g; fat: 5.2 g; calories: 62.

Macronutrient ratio: calories from carbs: 16 percent; protein: 12 percent; fat: 73 percent.

Squash Chips

Squash is high in antioxidants and vitamin C and a good source of manganese, a mineral that helps the body process fats, carbohydrates, and glucose. This chip will squash any traditional packaged "chip" out there.

3 medium yellow squash or zucchini

Coconut oil spray or regular coconut oil

Dash of salt

Dash of garlic powder

Dash of Parmesan cheese (optional)

1. Preheat the oven to 450°F (230°C, or gas mark 8). Grease or spray a baking sheet with coconut oil.

2. Slice the squash into thin chips of a consistent thickness. A mandolin slicer will help greatly here.

3. Lay the squash flat on the baking sheet. Coat the squash chips with oil. Sprinkle the salt, garlic powder, and cheese, if desired.

4. Bake for about 10 minutes, or until they start to brown, and then turn the chips. Bake for an additional 5 minutes, or until they start to brown. Turn off the heat and let the chips sit in the oven for an hour.

5. Check on them periodically so they don't burn. Letting them sit will help them to crisp, but if you don't have time to wait, just bake them an additional 5 to 7 minutes until they are brown.

YIELD: 4 servings

....

NUTRITIONAL FACTS

Per serving (5 oz, or 148 g): total carbs: 4.6 g; fiber: 1.3 g; net carbs: 3.3 g; protein: 1.8 g; fat: 0.5 g; calories: 25.

Macronutrient ratio: calories from carbs: 62 percent; protein: 24 percent; fat: 14 percent.

Zesty Walnut Brussels Sprouts

These brussels sprouts will please just about anyone's taste buds, thanks to a zing from the lemon juice. Be sure to make enough for leftovers, because they soak in flavor over time and are even better the next day.

½ cup (60 g) walnuts, chopped

1 pound (455 g) brussels sprouts, halved or quartered

2 to 3 tablespoons (27 to 40 g) coconut oil, melted

½ teaspoon salt

Ground black pepper, to taste

2 tablespoons (28 ml) extra-virgin olive oil

Juice from ½ of a lemon

1. Preheat the oven to 350°F (180°C, or gas mark 4). Scatter the walnuts on a baking sheet and bake for 10 minutes, or until toasted and fragrant. Set aside to cool.

2. Increase the oven to 400°F (200°C, or gas mark 6). Line a baking sheet with parchment paper.

3. In a medium bowl, toss together the brussels sprouts, coconut oil, salt, and pepper. Lay the sprouts out on the prepared baking sheet and roast for 35 minutes, or until fork-tender. Stir them halfway through baking to help them cook evenly.

4. Place the sprouts in a bowl and mix in the walnuts, olive oil, and lemon juice.

5. Store any leftovers in the fridge and then eat cool or warm briefly in the microwave or a pan.

YIELD: 4 to 6 servings

....
NUTRITIONAL FACTS

Per serving, for 4 (5 oz, or 146 g): total carbs: 12.3 g; fiber: 5.2 g; net carbs: 7.1 g; protein: 5.8 g; fat: 22.2 g; calories: 252.

Per serving, for 6 (3.5 oz, or 98 g): total carbs: 8.2 g; fiber: 3.4 g; net carbs: 4.7 g; protein: 3.8 g; fat: 14.8 g; calories: 168.

Macronutrient ratio: calories from carbs: 18 percent; protein: 9 percent; fat: 74 percent.

Green Deviled Eggs & Bacon

These scrambled eggs with avocado and a side of bacon will become one of your favorite breakfasts. These are a great way to have that yummy, healthy breakfast as a fun, handheld snack.

4 slices nitrite-free bacon

4 eggs

1 ripe avocado

2 teaspoons (10 ml) hot sauce

Juice from ¼ lime

¼ teaspoon salt

Dash of garlic powder

Dash of smoked paprika for topping (optional)

1. Preheat the oven to 375°F (190°C, or gas mark 5). Line a baking sheet with aluminum foil. Set the bacon on a baking rack, if you have one, on the baking sheet and bake for 10 minutes on each side.

2. Meanwhile, place the eggs in a saucepan and cover them by 1 to 2 inches (2.5 to 5 cm) of cold water. Bring the water to a boil over high heat, and then remove the pan from the heat, cover, and let sit for 12 minutes. Pour out the hot water and replace with cold.

3. While the eggs and bacon are cooking, in a small bowl, combine the avocado, hot sauce, lime juice, salt, and garlic powder. Mix until fairly smooth.

4. When the eggs are cold, peel them and cut in half lengthwise. Gently remove the yolk (rinse if necessary, and place face-down on a paper towel to dry). Spoon the avocado mixture into the yolk hole. If you want to make it look pretty, cut about ¼ inch (6.5 mm) from the bottom corner of a sandwich bag, put the avocado mixture in, and squeeze it into the eggs.

5. Once the bacon has cooled, pat off the grease, crumble into bits, and add to the top of the avocado-filled eggs. Sprinkle paprika on top, if desired.

YIELD: 4 servings

NUTRITIONAL FACTS

Per serving (1 egg): total carbs: 3.6 g; fiber: 2.3 g; net carbs: 1.2 g; protein: 10 g; fat: 12.5 g; calories: 164.

Macronutrient ratio: calories from carbs: 9 percent; protein: 24 percent; fat: 68 percent.

Avocado-Stuffed Eggs

These are best made just before eating to avoid the avocado turning brown. If you'd like to be a little more decorative, top with a slice of ripe olive, a little minced cilantro, or both.

12 large eggs, hard boiled

2 ripe avocados

2 tablespoons (28 g) mayonnaise

2 tablespoons (20 g) minced red onion

1 tablespoon (15 ml) lime juice

½ clove of garlic, crushed

¼ teaspoon salt, or as needed

½ teaspoon Tabasco Chipotle sauce

Paprika, for garnish

Sliced ripe olives, for garnish

Minced fresh cilantro, for garnish

1. Peel the eggs and slice them in half, turning the yolks out into a food processor bowl. Set the whites aside.

2. Slice the avocados in half, remove the pits, scoop the innards of one avocado into the processor with the yolks, and add the mayo. Process, scraping down the sides as needed, until smooth.

3. Scrape into a bowl and add the flesh of the other avocado. Mash it in roughly—a whisk is good for this. Add the minced onion, lime juice, garlic, salt, and Tabasco and mash them in, too. Stuff the yolk-avocado mixture into the whites.

4. Sprinkle the eggs with paprika.

YIELD: 24 servings

....

NUTRITIONAL FACTS

Per serving (½ egg): total carbs: 1.4 g; fiber: 0.8 g; net carbs: 0.6 g; protein: 3.4 g; fat: 5.3 g; calories: 66.

Macronutrient ratio: calories from carbs: 9 percent; protein: 20 percent; fat: 71 percent.

Caesar Eggs

One of our testers said this recipe took 20 minutes, rated it a 10, and added, "We ate a lot of them and spoiled our dinner." It doesn't matter—these make a perfectly fine dinner, as well as lunch or a snack.

12 large eggs, hard boiled

½ cup (115 g) mayonnaise

1 ½ tablespoons (23 g) brown mustard

2 teaspoons anchovy paste

1 ½ teaspoons lemon juice

½ teaspoon Worcestershire sauce

¼ cup (25 g) Parmesan cheese

2 tablespoons (8 g) minced fresh parsley

1. Peel the eggs and halve them, turning the yolks out into a food processor. Set aside the whites. Add the mayonnaise, mustard, anchovy paste, lemon juice, and Worcestershire sauce to the yolks. Run the processor until the mixture is very smooth.

2. Stuff this mixture into the whites. Sprinkle the eggs with the Parmesan and parsley, and serve, or refrigerate until party time.

YIELD: 24 servings

....

NUTRITIONAL FACTS

Per serving (½ egg): total carbs: 0.5 g; fiber: 0 g; net carbs: 0.5 g; protein: 3.6 g; fat: 6.4 g; calories: 76.

Macronutrient ratio: calories from carbs: 3 percent; protein: 19 percent; fat: 78 percent.

Prosciutto-Wrapped Asparagus

With just three simple ingredients, this supertasty snack is a great late afternoon treat. Serve it to your family and friends and before you know it, they'll all be gone . . . and that's a good thing!

1 pound (455 g) fresh asparagus

4 ounces (115 g) thinly sliced prosciutto

1 tablespoon (14 g) ghee or grass-fed butter

1. Cut the bottom 2 inches (5 cm) off the asparagus. Then cut each slice of prosciutto in half lengthwise and individually wrap each piece around an asparagus spear.

2. In a large skillet over medium-high heat, melt the ghee. Add the wrapped asparagus and cook for about 2 minutes on each side, until the prosciutto is crispy. Reduce the heat to low and cook for about 10 minutes so the asparagus can steam.

3. Alternatively, you can roast them at 450°F (230°C, or gas mark 8) on a baking sheet. After you've wrapped the asparagus with prosciutto, brush them with melted ghee/butter, bake for 5 minutes on one side, flip, and bake for an additional 5 minutes.

YIELD: 4 servings

NUTRITIONAL FACTS

Per serving: total carbs: 2.4 g; fiber: 1.2 g; net carbs: 1.2 g; protein: 9.2 g; fat: 5.6 g; calories: 95.

Macronutrient ratio: calories from carbs: 10 percent; protein: 38 percent; fat: 52 percent.

Cauliflower Hummus

Light and fluffy, this snack tastes even better than traditional hummus. It has all the wonderful flavors of a Greek snack, but without the difficult-to-digest legumes.

1 medium head of cauliflower (about 2 cups [200 g] florets)

1/3 cup (80 g) tahini

1/4 cup (60 ml) fresh lemon juice

2 tablespoons (28 ml) extra-virgin olive oil

1 clove of garlic

3/4 teaspoon salt

Ground black pepper, to taste

Dash of smoked paprika (optional)

1. Place a steamer basket in a medium pot and fill the pot with about 2 inches (5 cm) of water. If you don't have a basket, use a colander on top of your pot. Bring the water to a boil. Place the cauliflower florets in the steamer basket or colander. Cover and allow the florets to steam for 8 minutes, or until soft.

2. Transfer the cauliflower to a food processor. Add the tahini, lemon juice, olive oil, garlic, salt, and pepper. Blend until smooth. That's it! Dust with smoked paprika, if desired, before serving.

3. This hummus goes great with My Favorite Crunchy Crackers (page 106) or with any sliced raw veggies.

YIELD: 4 to 6 servings

NUTRITIONAL FACTS

Per serving, for 4 (6.75 oz, or 191 g): total carbs: 12.9 g; fiber: 3.9 g; net carbs: 9 g; protein: 6.4 g; fat: 18.1 g; calories: 220.

Per serving, for 6 (4.5 oz, or 127 g): total carbs: 8.6 g; fiber: 2.6 g; net carbs: 6 g; protein: 4.3 g; fat: 12 g; calories: 146.

Macronutrient ratio: calories from carbs: 22 percent; protein: 11 percent; fat: 68 percent.

Peanut Hummus

Hummus is a hugely popular snack, but this low-carb version replaces the chickpeas with peanuts. This is a little tricky to prepare, but it makes a lot and you can freeze it, so it's worth the extra time. It's awfully good with cut-up veggies! You can serve pita wedges or chips for your friends, if you like.

12 ounces (340 g) raw shelled peanuts

3/4 cup (175 ml) lemon juice (about 3 lemons)

2/3 cup (160 g) tahini

4 cloves of garlic, crushed (more or less, depending on how big they are and how garlicky you like your hummus)

1/3 cup (80 ml) extra-virgin olive oil, plus more for serving

1 teaspoon ground cumin

1/3 cup (80 ml) water, or as needed

Salt, to taste

1/4 cup (15 g) minced fresh parsley

Paprika, for garnish

1. Start by peeling the skins off the peanuts. (If you can get raw peanuts without the skins, grab 'em! If you're down South and can buy canned, boiled peanuts, this will be a snap.) Put the peanuts in a big saucepan, cover with water, and bring to a boil. All of 3 minutes later, remove them from the heat and drain. This will loosen the skins, and most of them will come off with rubbing. The more diligent you are about peeling your peanuts, the creamier your hummus will be.

2. Cover them with water again, bring to a boil, and then turn down the heat and simmer for a good 3 to 4 hours until they're soft like any cooked legume, which is, of course, what they are. Drain them again. (You can do this ahead of time and stash them in a snap-top container in the fridge for up to 5 days.)

3. To make the hummus, put the lemon juice and tahini in a food processor. Process these two ingredients for 4 to 5 minutes. This apparently does something magical to improve the texture of the hummus.

4. Add the boiled peanuts, garlic, olive oil, and cumin. Run the processor until the whole mixture is finely ground. Now blend in the water; use a little more or less water to get the texture you like.

5. Season with salt and then quickly blend in the parsley. It's done! This recipe makes quite a lot, so if you're not having a party, scrape it into a snap-top container and store it in the fridge. You can freeze it, too.

6. When it's time to serve the hummus, spoon some into a dish, swirling it nicely. Dust it with a little paprika to make it look pretty and then pour some olive oil over the top.

▶ **Note:** Tahini is sesame butter. Look for it in the grocery store with Middle Eastern and Asian foods.

YIELD: 20 servings

NUTRITIONAL FACTS

Per serving (1.5 oz, or 43 g): total carbs: 5.4 g; fiber: 1.9 g; net carbs: 3.5 g; protein: 5.9 g; fat: 16.4 g; calories: 179.

Macronutrient ratio: calories from carbs: 11 percent; protein: 12 percent; fat: 77 percent.

Roasted Red Pepper Dip

We all know how vitamin C is great for the common cold, but did you also know that it helps protect us from the harmful effects of stress? Vitamin C allows the body to quickly clear out cortisol, a primary stress hormone that increases sugars in the bloodstream. It just so happens that red peppers are the second highest plant source of vitamin C, containing almost 300 percent of our daily vitamin C intake. Mix all of that into a divine-tasting dip and you've got a superb snack!

1 cup (100 g) shelled walnuts

1 teaspoon smoked paprika

½ teaspoon onion powder

½ teaspoon salt

1 jar (12 ounces, or 340 g) roasted red peppers, drained

1 clove of garlic, minced

2 tablespoons (28 ml) extra-virgin olive oil

2 teaspoons lemon juice

In a food processor, pulse the walnuts, paprika, onion powder, and salt until the walnuts are finely ground (like the consistency of hummus). Add the peppers, garlic, olive oil, and lemon juice and blend until completely smooth.

YIELD: about 4 servings

....

NUTRITIONAL FACTS

Per serving (3.5 oz, or 101 g): total carbs: 8.9 g; fiber: 4.3 g; net carbs: 4.6 g; protein: 4 g; fat: 23.4 g; calories: 250.

Macronutrient ratio: calories from carbs: 14 percent; protein: 6 percent; fat: 80 percent.

Flatbread "PB&J"

This supertasty roll-up will let you enjoy a sandwich-like snack without the guilt or worry of eating a high-carb, gluten-filled, high-glycemic bread. Great with sunflower seed butter and fresh, cut-up strawberries or the fruit of your choice, you'll never have to miss sandwich bread . . . or the peanut butter or jelly for that matter.

½ cup (56 g) coconut flour

2 tablespoons (16 g) psyllium husk powder

1 tablespoon (12 g) coconut palm sugar

1 teaspoon ground cinnamon

¼ cup (54 g) coconut oil

1 cup (235 ml) boiling water

⅓ cup (75 g) sunflower seed butter

10 strawberries, thinly sliced

1. Preheat the oven to 375°F (190°C, or gas mark 5). Line a baking sheet with parchment paper. In a medium bowl, mix together the coconut flour, psyllium husk powder, coconut palm sugar, and cinnamon. Add the coconut oil and hot water and stir it all together.

2. Spread the dough out on the lined baking sheet. With a rolling pin or glass, flatten out the dough as evenly as you can so it's about ½ inch (1.5 cm) thick. Bake 15 minutes, or until a toothpick inserted in the middle comes out clean. Then move to a cooling rack and allow to cool to room temperature.

3. Once the dough is cool, spread the sunflower seed butter and strawberries (or whatever fruit you would like). Then carefully roll the "bread" and slice, with a pizza cutter or knife, into 3 inch (7.5 cm) pieces.

YIELD: 5 sandwiches

NUTRITIONAL FACTS

Per sandwich: total carbs: 19.8 g; fiber: 9.3 g; net carbs: 10.5 g; protein: 4.7 g; fat: 21.9 g; calories: 286.

Macronutrient ratio: calories from carbs: 27 percent; protein: 6 percent; fat: 67 percent.

Pork Belly Fat Bombs

If you're lucky enough to have leftover pork belly, use it to make these snack-size fat bombs. They're meaty and filling and, because they're laced with mustard and horseradish, they also pack quite a kick!

5.3 ounces (150 g) cooked pork belly (see Note)

6 pancetta slices or 3 bacon slices (3.2 ounces, or 90 g), cut in half widthwise

¼ cup (55 g/1.9 oz) mayonnaise, preferably homemade

1 tablespoon (15 g/0.5 oz) Dijon mustard

1 tablespoon (15 g/0.5 oz) grated fresh horseradish

Salt and pepper, to taste

Crispy lettuce leaves, for serving (optional)

1. Preheat the oven to 375°F (190°C, or gas mark 5). Line a baking sheet with parchment paper. Lay the bacon slices flat on the parchment, leaving enough space between so they don't overlap. Place the sheet in the oven and cook for 10 to 15 minutes, or until crispy. The exact amount of cooking time depends on the thickness of the bacon slices. Remove from the oven and set aside to cool. Pour the bacon grease into a glass container and reserve for another use, such as frying eggs. When cool enough to handle, crumble the bacon into a dish and set aside.

2. Shred the pork belly in a bowl. Mix in the mayonnaise, mustard, and horseradish. Season with salt and pepper. Divide the mixture into six mounds. Top with the crumbled bacon and serve on top of crispy lettuce leaves (if using). Enjoy immediately or refrigerate in an airtight container for up to 5 days.

YIELD: 6 servings

NUTRITIONAL FACTS

Per serving: total carbs: 0.5 g; fiber: 0.2 g; net carbs: 0.3 g; protein: 5.8 g; fat: 26.4 g; energy: 263 kcal.

Macronutrient ratio: calories from carbs: 1 percent; protein: 9 percent; fat: 90 percent.

▶ If you need to cook the pork belly, preheat the oven to 400°F (200°C, or gas mark 6). Using a sharp knife, score the pork skin down to the meat. Make the cuts close together and try not to cut the meat. Place it in a deep roasting pan and into the preheated oven. Cook for 30 minutes. Reduce the temperature to 325°F (160°C, or gas mark 3), and cook for 1 hour, 30 minutes more. Finally, increase the temperature to 425°F (220°C, or gas mark 7), and cook for another 30 minutes. Remove from the oven and set aside to cool at room temperature.

Zesty Cheddar-Stuffed Celery

The filling in this recipe has a wonderful texture, but you could gild the lily with a little crumbled bacon or minced jalapeño on top, if you want to take the trouble.

1 pound (455 g) sharp Cheddar cheese, shredded

2 ounces (55 g) cream cheese, softened

4 tablespoons (55 g) butter, softened

2 tablespoons (28 ml) dry sherry

2 teaspoons prepared horseradish

1 teaspoon Worcestershire sauce

14 large celery ribs

Run the Cheddar, cream cheese, butter, sherry, horseradish, and Worcestershire sauce through a food processor until well combined and then (surprise, surprise) stuff the mixture into the celery. Cut into 2 to 3 inch (5 to 7.5 cm)-lengths to serve.

YIELD: 56 servings

....

NUTRITIONAL FACTS

Per serving: total carbs: 0.8 g; fiber: 0 g; net carbs: 0.6 g; protein: 2 g; fat: 3.9 g; calories: 47.

Macronutrient ratio: calories from carbs: 7 percent; protein: 17 percent; fat: 75 percent.

Cashew Chicken Dip

Scoop up this dip with veggies! It's great for a party, of course, but it also makes a good snack or lunch. It's versatile, too—try it in omelets. It is marvelous that way, especially with a little extra sriracha on top.

3/4 cup (105 g) diced cooked chicken

2 scallions

3/4 cup (175 g) mayonnaise

1/4 cup (60 g) sour cream

1 tablespoon (15 ml) soy sauce

1 teaspoon grated fresh ginger

1/2 teaspoon sesame oil

1/4 teaspoon sriracha sauce

1 clove of garlic, crushed

1/2 cup (70 g) roasted salted cashews

1. Put everything but the cashews in your food processor. Pulse until everything is finely chopped and blended.

2. Add the cashews and pulse just enough to chop them up and distribute them, but not to pulverize them. You want recognizable bits of cashew in your dip.

3. Serve! If you have leftovers, store in a snap-top container in the fridge, but keep in mind that the cashews will soften.

YIELD: 8 servings

NUTRITIONAL FACTS

Per serving (2 oz, or 56 g): total carbs: 3.8 g; fiber: 0.1 g; net carbs: 3.4 g; protein: 6 g; fat: 21.7 g; calories: 231.

Macronutrient ratio: calories from carbs: 7 percent; protein: 10 percent; fat: 83 percent.

N'Oatmeal Cookies

You might remember the irresistible, old-fashioned oatmeal raisin cookies made with Crisco, white flour, sugar, and oats. Fast-forward to these N'Oatmeal Cookies—healthwise, the antithesis of the old-fashioned variety, but tastewise, equally as good.

2 cups (200 g) almond meal

½ cup (96 g) coconut palm sugar

2 tablespoons (16 g) arrowroot powder

1 tablespoon (7 g) ground cinnamon

1 teaspoon salt

¾ teaspoon baking soda

4 eggs, room temperature

½ cup (112 g) grass-fed butter, melted

¼ cup (85 g) maple syrup

1 teaspoon vanilla extract

½ cup (50 g) raw walnuts, roughly chopped

½ cup (50 g) raw pecans, roughly chopped

½ cup (73 g) raw almonds, roughly chopped

½ cup (75 g) raisins

1. Preheat the oven to 350°F (180°C, or gas mark 4). Line a baking sheet with parchment paper.

2. In a small bowl, mix together the almond meal, coconut palm sugar, arrowroot, cinnamon, salt, and baking soda. In a medium bowl, beat the eggs and then mix in the butter, maple syrup, and vanilla. Pour the dry ingredients into the wet and combine well. Fold in the walnuts, pecans, almonds, and raisins.

3. Use your hands or a tablespoon to shape the dough into 2½ inch (6.5 cm) cookies. Bake for 8 to 10 minutes, or until set.

YIELD: about 18 cookies

....

NUTRITIONAL FACTS

Per cookie: total carbs: 17.3 g; fiber: 2.6 g; net carbs: 14.7 g; protein: 5.7 g; fat: 18.1 g; calories: 243.

Macronutrient ratio: calories from carbs: 27 percent; protein: 9 percent; fat: 64 percent.

Happy Birthday Cookie Cake

Fresh out of the oven, the outside is crispy, and the ooey-gooey middle will remind you of a traditional cookie cake.

2 cups (520 g) almond or cashew butter

4 eggs

1 cup (340 g) maple syrup

½ cup (112 g) grass-fed butter, melted

2 tablespoons (16 g) arrowroot powder

2 teaspoons (10 ml) vanilla extract

1 teaspoon baking soda

½ teaspoon salt

1 cup (175 g) plus 1 cup (optional) dark chocolate chips, divided

1. Preheat the oven to 325°F (170°C, or gas mark 3). Grease an 8 x 13 inch (20 x 33 cm)-baking dish or 9 inch (23 cm)-pie plate.

2. In a medium bowl, combine the almond butter, eggs, maple syrup, butter, arrowroot powder, vanilla, baking soda, and salt with a hand mixer or fork. Then fold in 1 cup (175 g) of the chocolate chips. Pour the batter into the prepared pan, and bake for 35 to 50 minutes. If you want it a little gooey in the middle, cook it for 35 minutes. If you want it a little more firm and crispy, cook it for about 50 minutes, or until a toothpick inserted in the middle comes out clean.

3. To add the optional chocolate topping, in a medium heat-safe bowl, add 1 cup (175 g) chocolate chips and set the bowl over a saucepan of simmering water. Let the chocolate melt. Before the chocolate is completely melted, remove the bowl from the heat and stir the chocolate until it is smooth. Spread over the cake, let cool for about 10 minutes, and enjoy.

YIELD: 10 to 12 servings

....

NUTRITIONAL FACTS

Per serving, for 10: total carbs: 47.2 g; fiber: 5.3 g; net carbs: 40.3 g; protein: 15 g; fat: 46.8 g; calories: 628.

Per serving, for 12: total carbs: 39.3 g; fiber: 4.4 g; net carbs: 33.5 g; protein: 12.5 g; fat: 39 g; calories: 524.

Macronutrient ratio: calories from carbs: 28 percent; protein: 9 percent; fat: 63 percent.

Cannoli Pudding

This pudding has all of the rich goodness of a cannoli except without the pastry shell. It's creamy, delicious, and low-carb.

1 cup (240 g) mascarpone cheese

1 cup (250 g) full-fat ricotta cheese

36 drops liquid stevia (vanilla flavor)

1 tablespoon (15 ml) lemon juice

¼ teaspoon orange extract

½ teaspoon vanilla extract

2 tablespoons (15 g) raw, unsalted, shelled pistachio nuts

¼ ounce (7 g) 85 percent dark chocolate

1. Put both cheeses, the stevia, lemon juice, orange extract, and vanilla extract in a medium-size bowl and whip with an electric mixer for 3 to 4 minutes, until light and fluffy. Spoon into little dishes; the servings are small because it's so rich. At this point, you can refrigerate the pudding for several hours if you like.

2. Sometime before serving, preheat the oven to 350°F (180°C, or gas mark 4). Spread the pistachios on a small baking sheet and bake for 6 to 7 minutes. Chop them medium-fine. Again, you can do this ahead of time, if desired.

3. Just before serving, grate the chocolate over the individual servings of pudding. A Microplane grater works perfectly. (If using a box grater, grate the chocolate onto a sheet of waxed paper and then transfer to the puddings.) Top each with chopped pistachios and serve.

YIELD: 4 servings

....

NUTRITIONAL FACTS

Per serving (6.5 oz, or 185 g): total carbs: 4 g; fiber: 0.4 g; net carbs: 3.4 g; protein: 15.9 g; fat: 62.7 g; calories: 625.

Macronutrient ratio: calories from carbs: 3 percent; protein: 10 percent; fat: 87 percent.

Vanilla-Keto Ice Cream

*This low-carb ice cream is a scoopable fat bomb—and it's so ridicu-
lously rich and creamy that you'll mistake it for frozen vanilla custard.*

1½ cups (360 g/12.7 oz) creamed
coconut milk

6 large egg yolks

2 large eggs

¼ cup (40 g/1.4 oz) erythritol or
Swerve, powdered

¼ cup (60 ml /2 fl oz) MCT oil

2 teaspoons sugar-free vanilla extract
or 1 teaspoon vanilla powder

Few drops liquid stevia, to taste
(optional)

1. Make the creamed coconut milk a day ahead (see box for instructions).

2. In a food processor, combine the creamed coconut milk, egg yolks, eggs,
   erythritol, MCT oil, and vanilla. Pulse until smooth and creamy. If you want
   a sweeter taste, add the stevia and pulse again.

3. Pour the mixture into an ice cream maker and process according to the
   manufacturer's instructions. Once the ice cream is churned, freeze for about
   30 minutes before serving. Keep frozen for up to 3 months.

YIELD: 8 servings/scoops

....

NUTRITIONAL FACTS

Per serving (1 scoop [1/3 cup/85 g/3 oz]): total carbs: 3.9 g; fiber: 1 g; net carbs: 2.9 g;
protein: 5.2 g; fat: 27.1 g; energy: 270 kcal.

Macronutrient ratio: calories from carbs: 4 percent; protein: 8 percent; fat: 88 percent.

▶ **How to Make Creamed Coconut Milk**

Creamed coconut milk or coconut cream is the fatty part of coconut milk that has
been separated from the watery part. If a recipe calls for creamed coconut milk,
make it a day ahead. To "cream" coconut milk, simply place the can in the refrigerator
overnight. The next day, open the can, spoon out the solidified coconut milk, and
discard the liquids. Do not shake the can before opening. One 14 ounce (400 g)-can
will yield about 7 ounces (200 g) of coconut cream.

4

ON-THE-GO SNACKS:
Fun and Convenient for Commutes, Carpools, and Road Trips

We spend a great deal of our lives in the car. It's a necessary part of life. Whether you are going to work, carpooling to a child's activity, or heading out on a fun road trip, choosing the right snacks can be challenging. What can you bring that is fun, portable, tasty, easy to eat, keeps well, and of course, actually good for you?

Unfortunately, many prepackaged snacks are laden with preservatives and food coloring that, according to recent research by the UK's government-sponsored Food Commission, can increase temper tantrums and irritable behavior.

Fortunately for you, this chapter contains delicious snacks that are both fun and easy to eat—no spoon feeding or face wiping of little ones. They're made with no artificial colors, additives, or processed sugar. Even better, because they're low-glycemic, they will keep blood sugar levels stable.

Moreover, all these snacks fit neatly into sandwich bags or small storage containers, making them superportable.

Crispy Maple Granola

There is something about a sweet, salty, crunchy, and buttery treat all wrapped into one snack that is amazing. Add to that the health benefits of the grass-fed butter, which include immune-boosting, cancer-fighting, fat-burning nutrients. Also loaded with fiber, omega-3s, and other healthy fats, this snack is great for a car ride as it will keep you satiated a long time, or even at home with berries and almond or coconut milk.

3/4 cup (75 g) raw pecans

1/2 cup (73 g) raw almonds

1/2 cup (50 g) raw walnuts

3/4 cup (60 g) unsweetened shredded coconut

3 tablespoons (30 g) chia seeds

1/4 cup (85 g) maple syrup

2 1/2 tablespoons (35 g) grass-fed butter

1 1/2 teaspoons vanilla extract

1/4 teaspoon salt

1. Preheat the oven to 325°F (170°C, or gas mark 3). Line a baking sheet with parchment paper.

2. In a food processor, pulse the pecans, almonds, and walnuts into small pieces. Pour into a medium bowl with the shredded coconut and chia seeds; toss to combine. In a small saucepan, over medium-low heat, cook the maple syrup, butter, vanilla, and salt until it starts to bubble. Pour the liquid mixture over the nuts, coconut, and seeds. Mix well.

3. Spread onto the prepared baking sheet so it's not overlapping too much. Bake for 20 minutes, or until it starts to turn golden brown, tossing a couple of times so it cooks evenly. Once it comes out and starts to cool, it will get crunchier.

YIELD: 3 cups (366 g)

....

NUTRITIONAL FACTS

Per 1/4-cup serving (1 oz, or 34 g): total carbs: 9.5 g; fiber: 3 g; net carbs: 6.5 g; protein: 3.2 g; fat: 16.8 g; calories: 194.

Macronutrient ratio: calories from carbs: 19 percent; protein: 6 percent; fat: 75 percent.

Coconut Flapjacks

These easy, chewy cookie bars are a low-carb, grain-free take on an old English standard. They are homey and irresistible.

3/4 cup (165 g) butter

2 tablespoons (40 g) sugar-free imitation honey

1/4 cup (60 g) granular erythritol

1 cup (80 g) unsweetened shredded coconut

1 cup (112 g) flaxseed meal

1/4 teaspoon salt

1/4 teaspoon liquid stevia (English toffee flavor)

1. Preheat the oven to 350°F (180°C, or gas mark 4). Line a jelly roll pan with baking parchment.

2. In a small saucepan over low heat, melt the butter, imitation honey, and erythritol together.

3. In the meantime, add the coconut, flaxseed meal, and salt to a medium bowl and whisk together.

4. When the butter mixture is bubbling, whisk in the stevia. Then pour into the coconut-flax mixture and stir until everything is evenly coated.

5. Turn this soft, sticky dough out onto the parchment-lined baking pan, spread, and press it out to cover the whole pan evenly.

6. Bake for 15 to 18 minutes or until evenly golden. Immediately cut into bars while hot. Leave them in the baking pan until completely cool and then store in a snap-top container.

YIELD: 32 servings

....

NUTRITIONAL FACTS

Per serving (1/2 oz, or 14 g): total carbs: 4.5 g; fiber: 1.3 g; net carbs: 0.7 g; protein: 1 g; fat: 6.9 g; calories: 73.

Macronutrient ratio: calories from carbs: 22 percent; protein: 5 percent; fat: 74 percent.

Cinnamon Raisin Bars

Reminiscent of old-school cinnamon raisin bread, this delicious and easy-to-eat snack is perfect for the car. It can also be made nut-free by substituting the almond butter with a sunflower seed butter and leaving out the walnuts (or substituting with dark chocolate chips).

4 eggs

1 cup (260 g) almond butter or sunflower seed butter

1/3 cup (115 g) maple syrup

2 tablespoons (28 g) grass-fed butter, melted

2 tablespoons (24 g) coconut palm sugar

2 tablespoons (14 g) ground cinnamon

1 teaspoon vanilla extract

1/2 teaspoon baking soda

1/2 teaspoon salt

1/4 cup (35 g) raisins or currants

1/4 cup (25 g) walnuts (optional)

1. Preheat the oven to 325°F (170°C, or gas mark 3). Grease an 8 x 8-inch (20 x 20-cm) baking dish with coconut oil or palm shortening.

2. In a large bowl, combine the eggs, almond butter, maple syrup, butter, coconut palm sugar, cinnamon, vanilla, baking soda, and salt and stir until smooth. Fold in the raisins and walnuts, if using. Pour the batter into the prepared baking dish and move the dish around to ensure the batter is even. Bake for 25 minutes, or until a toothpick inserted in the middle of the bars comes out clean. Allow to cool for 30 minutes before cutting into bars and enjoying.

YIELD: 16 bars

NUTRITIONAL FACTS

Per serving, w/o walnuts: total carbs: 11.9 g; fiber: 2.3 g; net carbs: 9.7 g; protein: 5.1 g; fat: 11.6 g; calories: 163.

Macronutrient ratio: calories from carbs: 28 percent; protein: 12 percent; fat: 60 percent.

Per serving, w/ walnuts: total carbs: 12.2 g; fiber: 2.4 g; net carbs: 9.8 g; protein: 5.3 g; fat: 12.6 g; calories: 174.

Macronutrient ratio: calories from carbs: 26 percent; protein: 12 percent; fat: 62 percent.

Mini Zucchini Muffins

These fun, supertasty, and easy-to-eat mini muffins are like little shots of omega-3s for your brain. Studies have shown omega-3s can increase happiness and relaxation. Who couldn't use a little more of that while on the road?

1 cup (112 g) almond flour

1 cup (128 g) flaxseed meal

⅓ cup (64 g) coconut palm sugar

1½ teaspoons ground cinnamon

½ teaspoon salt

½ teaspoon baking soda

2 eggs

¼ cup (55 g) grass-fed butter, melted

½ cup (60 g) chopped raw walnuts

⅓ cup (50 g) currants or raisins

1 cup (124 g) peeled and grated zucchini (about 2 medium)

1. Preheat the oven to 350°F (180°C, or gas mark 4). Grease a mini-muffin pan.

2. In a medium bowl, mix the almond flour, flaxseed meal, coconut palm sugar, cinnamon, salt, and baking soda. In a small bowl, beat the eggs, and then add the melted butter, walnuts, and raisins. Add the wet ingredients to the dry and mix until well blended. Then mix in the zucchini until combined.

3. Scoop the batter into the prepared muffin cups about they are three-quarters full. Bake for 25 minutes, or until a toothpick inserted in the middle of a muffin comes out clean.

YIELD: 32 mini muffins

....

NUTRITIONAL FACTS

Per muffin: total carbs: 5.6 g; fiber: 1.6 g; net carbs: 3.9 g; protein: 2.3 g; fat: 5.4 g; calories: 75.

Macronutrient ratio: calories from carbs: 28 percent; protein: 11 percent; fat: 61 percent.

Chocolate Chip Muffins

These moist and delicious little snacks will not only satisfy your taste buds but will keep you feeling full thanks to an abundance of healthy fats. Because they are made with low-glycemic sweeteners and a little caffeine (thank you, chocolate), these muffins will recharge your batteries—without the big sugar spike and fall associated with most sweet snacks. Try to set your eggs out ahead of time so they can warm to room temperature. Otherwise, the chill from the eggs will solidify the coconut oil and can make the batter clumpy.

3 eggs, room temperature

½ teaspoon vanilla extract

1 cup (260 g) almond butter

1 cup (112 g) almond flour

½ cup (96 g) coconut palm sugar

⅓ cup (72 g) coconut oil, melted

½ teaspoon baking soda

¼ teaspoon salt

½ cup (88 g) dark chocolate chips

1. Preheat the oven to 350°F (180°C, or gas mark 4). Line a 12-cup muffin pan with silicone or paper muffin liners, or grease the cups.

2. In a small bowl, beat the eggs and then add the vanilla. In a medium bowl, mix together the almond butter, almond flour, coconut palm sugar, coconut oil, baking soda, and salt. Add the egg mixture and stir until well combined. Fold in the chocolate chips.

3. Pour the batter into the prepared muffin cups until about two-thirds full. Bake for 20 minutes, or until a toothpick inserted in the middle of a muffin comes out clean. Cool slightly before removing muffins from pan.

YIELD: 12 muffins

....

NUTRITIONAL FACTS

Per muffin: total carbs: 20.1 g; fiber: 3.2 g; net carbs: 16.3 g; protein: 8.7 g; fat: 26.7 g; calories: 333.

Macronutrient ratio: calories from carbs: 23 percent; protein: 10 percent; fat: 68 percent.

Rich and Tender Crackers

The name says it all. These versatile crackers have a tender, buttery crunch.

1 cup (145 g) raw sunflower seeds

½ cup (65 g) rice protein powder

2 teaspoons xanthan

½ teaspoon baking powder

½ teaspoon salt, plus more for sprinkling

4 tablespoons (55 g) butter, softened

1 egg white

1 tablespoon (15 ml) water

1. Preheat the oven to 350°F (180°C, or gas mark 4).

2. Put the sunflower seeds, rice protein powder, xanthan, baking powder, and salt in a food processor, and run it until the whole thing becomes a fine, even meal.

3. Add the butter and run the processor until well incorporated. Add the egg white and again run until it's incorporated. Finally, add the water and run until you have a soft dough.

4. Line a cookie sheet with baking parchment. Make a ball of half the dough and place in the middle of the parchment. Cover with another sheet of parchment and, with a rolling pin, roll out into as thin and even a sheet as you can. Peel off the top sheet of parchment. Using a thin, sharp, straight-bladed knife, score the dough into squares, diamonds, or triangles.

5. Bake for 25 minutes or until golden. While they're baking, roll out and cut the rest of the dough on a second cookie sheet. When the first batch is done, bake the second.

6. Cool on the cookie sheets, re-score to break apart, and store in a snap-top container.

YIELD: 50 servings

....

NUTRITIONAL FACTS

Per cracker (1/4 oz, or 6 g): total carbs: 0.8 g; fiber: 0.2 g; net carbs: 0.4 g; protein: 1.6 g; fat: 2.4 g; calories: 30.

Macronutrient ratio: calories from carbs: 10 percent; protein: 21 percent; fat: 69 percent.

Anchovy-Olive Crackers

Using sunflower seed kernels instead of the wheat flour in the original recipe produced a worthy low-carb alternative.

1½ cups (218 g) sunflower seeds

½ teaspoon baking powder

½ teaspoon xanthan or guar

½ cup (50 g) grated Parmesan or Romano cheese, or a combination

8 anchovy fillets packed in olive oil

3 tablespoons (19 g) chopped black olives

1 tablespoon (15 ml) water

Salt, to taste

1. Preheat the oven to 350°F (180°C, or gas mark 4).

2. Put the sunflower seeds, baking powder, and xanthan or guar in a food processor and run it until the seeds are a fine meal.

3. Add the Parmesan and anchovy fillets and run the processor until the anchovies are pulverized and completely incorporated.

4. Add the olives and water. Pulse just enough to combine; you want flecks of olive to be visible in the finished crackers.

5. Line a cookie sheet with baking parchment. Make a ball of half the dough and place in the middle of the parchment. Cover with another sheet of parchment and, using a rolling pin, roll into as thin and even a sheet as you can. Peel off the top parchment, sprinkle the dough with salt, and then use a sharp, thin, straight-bladed knife to score into squares, diamonds, or triangles.

6. Bake for 25 minutes or until golden. While they're baking, roll out and cut the rest of the dough on a second cookie sheet. When the first batch is done, bake the second.

7. Cool on the cookie sheet, re-score to break apart, and store in a snap-top container.

YIELD: About 50 crackers

....

NUTRITIONAL FACTS

Per cracker (1/4 oz, or 6 g): total carbs: 1 g; fiber: 0.4 g; net carbs: 0.6 g; protein: 1.2 g; fat: 2.5 g; calories: 29.

Macronutrient ratio: calories from carbs: 13 percent; protein: 15 percent; fat: 72 percent.

Favorite Crackers

There is no better name for this cracker. Low-glycemic and full of protein, with good fats including lots of omega-3s, this easy-to-eat snack is ideal for in the car, or anywhere else for that matter.

1 cup (112 g) almond flour

½ cup (64 g) flaxseed meal

½ cup (92 g) chia seeds

1¼ teaspoons (7.5 g) salt

2 teaspoons (3 g) Italian seasoning

1 teaspoon garlic powder

1 egg

2 tablespoons (28 ml) extra-virgin olive oil

1. Preheat the oven to 350°F (180°C, or gas mark 4).

2. In a medium bowl, combine the almond flour, flaxseed meal, chia seeds, salt, Italian seasoning, garlic powder, and mix well. Add the egg and olive oil and stir until a dough forms.

3. Place half of the dough on a piece of parchment paper. Top with another piece of parchment paper and roll with rolling pin to about ⅛ inch (3 mm) thick. Remove the top piece of parchment. With a pizza cutter, score individual crackers into squares. Transfer the dough and bottom piece of parchment to a baking sheet. Bake for 8 minutes, or until they start to turn brown. Then turn off the heat and let them sit in the oven for another 10 minutes or so.

4. Once those are done, you can lay out the second batch on the prepared baking sheet and begin baking them. You can also bake them on two baking sheets, one on each rack in the oven; just shuffle the baking sheets halfway through the bake time.

YIELD: about 50 crackers

....

NUTRITIONAL FACTS

Per cracker (1/4 oz, or 7 g): total carbs: 1.6 g; fiber: 1.1 g; net carbs: 0.5 g; protein: 1.1 g; fat: 2.6 g; calories: 32.

Macronutrient ratio: calories from carbs: 19 percent; protein: 13 percent; fat: 68 percent.

Rosemary-Cheese Crackers

The flavor combination is irresistible and using ground sunflower seed kernels instead of flour makes these a delicious, low-carb delight.

1 cup (145 g) sunflower seeds

½ cup (65 g) rice protein powder

½ teaspoon xanthan or guar

½ teaspoon baking powder

½ teaspoon salt, plus more for sprinkling

2 tablespoons (28 g) butter, softened

1½ tablespoons (3 g) minced fresh rosemary

1 cup (115 g) shredded sharp Cheddar cheese

½ cup (50 g) shredded Parmesan cheese

1 egg white

3 tablespoons (45 ml) water

1. Preheat the oven to 350°F (180°C, or gas mark 4).

2. Put the sunflower seeds, rice protein powder, xanthan or guar, baking powder, and salt in a food processor and run it until the sunflower seeds are ground up to the texture of cornmeal or finer.

3. With the processor running, add the butter and rosemary. Then work in the cheeses in three or four additions. Add the egg white and then the water. When it forms a soft dough, turn off the processor.

4. Line a cookie sheet with parchment. Make a ball of half the dough, put it on the parchment, and then put another sheet of parchment over it. Use a rolling pin to roll the dough out into as thin and even a sheet as you can. Carefully peel off the top sheet of parchment. Using a thin, sharp, straight-bladed knife, score the dough into crackers. Sprinkle them lightly with salt.

5. Bake for 20 to 25 minutes or until golden. While they're baking, roll out and cut the rest of the dough on a second cookie sheet. When the first batch is done, bake the second. Cool on the cookie sheets, re-score to break apart, and store in a snap-top container.

YIELD: About 50 crackers

....
NUTRITIONAL FACTS

Per cracker (1/3 oz, or 9 g): total carbs: 0.8 g; fiber: 0.3 g; net carbs: 0.5 g; protein: 2.5 g; fat: 2.9 g; calories: 38.

Macronutrient ratio: calories from carbs: 8 percent; protein: 25 percent; fat: 67 percent.

Chile-Lime Peanuts

Crunchy, a little spicy, with a Southwestern kick, these are supertasty—and superportable!

12 ounces (340 g) raw, shelled peanuts

1½ tablespoons (21 g) coconut oil, melted

1 tablespoon (15 ml) lime juice

½ teaspoon pure ground chile powder

½ teaspoon paprika (Smoked paprika is great, but use what you have.)

⅛ teaspoon cayenne pepper

Salt, to taste

1. Preheat the oven to 350°F (180°C, or gas mark 4). Line a jelly roll pan with aluminum foil.

2. Dump the peanuts onto the pan.

3. In a small dish, mix together the coconut oil, lime juice, chile powder, paprika, and cayenne.

4. Slowly pour the seasoning mixture over the peanuts, stirring the nuts constantly. Make sure they're all evenly coated.

5. Put them in the oven and set the timer for 5 minutes. When it beeps, remove and stir them again and return to the oven for another 5 minutes. Stir again, return to the oven, and give them a final 5 minutes.

6. Sprinkle with salt and let cool. Store in a tightly lidded container.

▶ **Note:** Look around your grocery stores for peanuts in bulk, which are often cheaper than the packaged variety.

YIELD: 12 servings

NUTRITIONAL FACTS

Per serving (1 oz, or 32 g): total carbs: 4.8 g; fiber: 2.5 g; net carbs: 2.3 g; protein: 7.4 g; fat: 15.7 g; calories: 177.

Macronutrient ratio: calories from carbs: 10 percent; protein: 16 percent; fat: 74 percent.

Spicy Pumpkin Seeds

Pumpkin seeds are a terrific source of minerals. They are cheaper than nuts, too. So here's something simple and savory to do with them in this Louisiana-style recipe.

¼ cup (56 g) coconut oil

2 cups (454 g) raw shelled pumpkin seeds

4 teaspoons (12 g) Creole seasoning

1. Put a large skillet over medium-low heat and melt the coconut oil. Add the pumpkin seeds and stir until they puff a bit and start turning golden, about 5 to 6 minutes.

2. Stir in the Creole seasoning and remove from the heat. That's it!

▶ **Note:** Look for shelled pumpkin seeds in the bulk section of your health food store, or in Mexican markets, where they are labeled "pepitas."

YIELD: 8 servings

....

NUTRITIONAL FACTS

Per 1/4-cup serving (1.5 oz, or 40 g): total carbs: 3.5 g; fiber: 1.9 g; net carbs: 1.5 g; protein: 9.8 g; fat: 22.6 g; calories: 241.

Macronutrient ratio: calories from carbs: 5 percent; protein: 15 percent; fat: 79 percent.

Pumpkin Bars

These savory treats are perfectly sweet-ened. With a whole cup of pumpkin in the mix, this snack is full of fiber to keep you full, as well as vitamin A and iron to help keep your immune system strong.

1 cup (245 g) pumpkin purée

½ cup (130 g) almond butter

⅓ cup (64 g) coconut palm sugar

1 tablespoon (7 g) coconut flour

1 tablespoon (7 g) pumpkin pie spice

1 tablespoon (20 g) maple syrup

½ teaspoon vanilla extract

2 eggs

¼ teaspoon baking soda

⅛ teaspoon salt

Handful of walnuts, chopped (optional)

1. Preheat the oven to 350°F (180°C, or gas mark 4). Grease an 8 x 8-inch (20 x 20-cm) baking dish.

2. In a large bowl (or food processor), mix together the pumpkin purée, almond butter, palm sugar, coconut flour, pumpkin pie spice, maple syrup, vanilla, eggs, baking soda, and salt until well blended. Pour the mixture into the prepared baking dish. Bake for about 40 minutes, or until a toothpick inserted in the middle comes out clean. Allow to cool for about 30 minutes and then eat as is or top with chopped walnuts.

YIELD: 12 bars

....

NUTRITIONAL FACTS

Per bar: total carbs: 10.9 g; fiber: 2 g; net carbs: 8.9 g; protein: 3.6 g; fat: 6.9 g; calories: 113.

Macronutrient ratio: calories from carbs: 36 percent; protein: 12 percent; fat: 52 percent.

Spiced Walnuts

English walnuts meet Asian seasonings. Imagine yourself on the terrace of the famous Raffles Hotel in Singapore when you serve these.

2 cups (200 g) walnut halves

2 tablespoons (30 g) granular Swerve

18 drops liquid stevia (English toffee flavor)

1 tablespoon (15 ml) soy sauce

2 teaspoons coconut oil, melted

1/2 teaspoon sriracha sauce

1/2 teaspoon smoked paprika

1/8 teaspoon cayenne pepper

Salt, to taste

1. Preheat the oven to 325°F (170°C, or gas mark 3). Line a jelly roll pan with baking parchment.

2. Put the walnuts in a medium-size bowl. In a custard cup, mix together every-thing else but the salt. Pour this over the walnuts and stir until they're evenly coated. Spread the nuts on the baking parchment in a single layer.

3. Put them in the oven and set the timer for 5 minutes. When it beeps, stir the nuts, spread them out again, and give them 5 minutes more. Stir again, spread them out again, and give them a final 5 minutes.

4. When they're crisp, remove from the oven, season them lightly with salt while they're still hot, and then let them cool on the parchment. Store in a snap-top container.

YIELD: 8 servings

....

NUTRITIONAL FACTS

Per 1/4-cup serving (1 oz, or 32 g): total carbs: 6.7 g; fiber: 1.7 g; net carbs: 5 g; protein: 4 g; fat: 17.5 g; calories: 176.

Macronutrient ratio: calories from carbs: 13 percent; protein: 8 percent; fat: 79 percent.

Mock Pâté

Celery stuffed with this yummy spread makes an easy, take-along snack or lunch. It also makes a great party food served with celery or low-carb crackers. It's good in omelets, too.

8 ounces (225 g) braunschweiger (liverwurst)

3 ounces (85 g) cream cheese, softened

¼ cup (60 ml) heavy cream

1 tablespoon (14 g) butter, melted

1 tablespoon (15 ml) Worcestershire sauce

Salt and ground black pepper, to taste

Just put everything in your food processor and run until it's well combined. Heap it in a small, pretty dish and serve with your choice of accompaniments.

YIELD: 6 servings

....

NUTRITIONAL FACTS

Per serving (2¹⁄3 oz, or 67 g): total carbs: 2.8 g; fiber: 0 g; net carbs: 2.8 g; protein: 6.7 g; fat: 21.2 g; calories: 226.

Macronutrient ratio: calories from carbs: 5 percent; protein: 12 percent; fat: 84 percent.

"Peanut Butter" Cookies

Sunflower seeds have a similar makeup to that of peanuts. When it comes to oil, protein, and carbohydrate contents, they're pretty close. The taste of these cookies is as close as you can get to a peanut butter cookie, and just as mouthwatering, but without the peanuts. Sunflower seeds also are considered to be one of the best whole-food sources of vitamin E, which helps protect brain cells and lowers the risk for chronic diseases. So now you have an excuse to eat even more of this rich, delectable treat!

2 cups (520 g) sunflower seed butter (16-ounce jar)

1 cup (192 g) coconut palm sugar

1 tablespoon (15 ml) vanilla extract

1/4 teaspoon salt

1. Preheat the oven to 350°F (180°C, or gas mark 4). Line a baking sheet with parchment paper.

2. In a medium bowl, mix together the sunflower seed butter, coconut palm sugar, vanilla extract, and salt and stir until well combined. Form golf ball–size pieces of dough and set on the prepared baking sheet. (Make sure the cookies have about 1 inch [2.5 cm] between them. You may have to use two baking sheets or bake in two batches.) Press the dough down to make the cookies a little flat and then use a fork to press a crisscross pattern onto them. Bake for 10 minutes, or until a toothpick inserted in the middle of a cookie comes out clean. (They will not turn brown on top like traditional peanut butter cookies.) Enjoy!

YIELD: about 24 cookies

....

NUTRITIONAL FACTS

Per cookie: total carbs: 13 g; fiber: 1.2 g; net carbs: 11.8 g; protein: 3.7 g; fat: 11.8 g; calories: 163.

Macronutrient ratio: calories from carbs: 30 percent; protein: 9 percent; fat: 61 percent.

Blonde Snack Bars

These moist, fluffy, and delicious bars taste like dessert! Because they are high in protein, have lots of healthy fat from the almond butter, and contain only low-glycemic sugars, they won't cause blood sugar swings or ramp up cravings like most traditional sweets or packaged snacks would.

2 cups (520 g) almond butter

6 eggs

1 cup (192 g) coconut palm sugar

4 teaspoons (20 ml) vanilla extract

1 teaspoon salt

1 teaspoon baking soda

1 cup (175 g) dark chocolate chips

1. Preheat the oven to 325°F (170°C, or gas mark 3). Grease a 9 x 13 inch (23 x 33 cm) baking dish or pan.

2. In a medium bowl, mix together the almond butter, eggs, coconut palm sugar, vanilla, salt, and baking soda. Fold in the chocolate chips. Spread the batter into the prepared dish and bake for 45 to 50 minutes, until a toothpick inserted in the middle comes out clean. Allow to cool for 10 minutes before cutting into bars.

3. To make these nut-free, you can use sunflower seed butter, but be aware that as the bars cool, the insides will turn green due to a chemical reaction with the baking soda. They are still totally fine and good to eat. Might be a great snack for St. Patrick's Day!

YIELD: 24 bars

NUTRITIONAL FACTS

Per bar: total carbs: 18.2 g; fiber: 2.2 g; net carbs: 15.3 g; protein: 6.7 g; fat: 16.1 g; calories: 228.

Macronutrient ratio: calories from carbs: 30 percent; protein: 11 percent; fat: 59 percent.

Almond Bliss Bars

Chocolate and coconut: it's like the perfect island wedding. Add almonds, and it's the perfect love triangle! These sugar-free bars are absolutely irresistible and make a great post-workout snack.

FOR BARS:

½ cup (120 g/4.2 oz) creamed coconut milk

1½ cups (112 g/4 oz) unsweetened shredded coconut

¼ cup (55 g/1.9 oz) coconut oil, at room temperature

2 tablespoons (20 g/0.7 oz) erythritol or Swerve, powdered

2 teaspoons sugar-free vanilla extract or 1 teaspoon vanilla powder

Pinch salt

Few drops liquid stevia, to taste (optional)

20 whole almonds (24 g/0.8 oz)

FOR COATING (or use any of the Homemade Dark Chocolate recipes [page 33]):

2 ounces (56 g) extra-dark 90 percent chocolate

0.8 ounces (24 g) cacao butter

1. To make creamed coconut milk, follow the instructions on page 93.

2. To make the bars: In a mixing bowl, stir together the creamed coconut milk, shredded coconut, coconut oil, erythritol, vanilla, and salt. If you want a sweeter taste, add the stevia and mix again. Use your hands to form the mixture into 10 small bars, about 1 ounce/(32 g) each, and place them on a parchment-lined tray. Top each bar with 2 almonds. Freeze for about 30 minutes.

3. To make the coating: Melt the dark chocolate in a double boiler, or heat-proof bowl placed over a small saucepan filled with 1 cup of water, over medium heat. Remove from the heat and set aside to cool.

4. Gently pierce each bar with a toothpick or a fork. Working one at a time, hold each bar over the melted dark chocolate and spoon the chocolate over it to coat completely. Turn the stick as you work until the coating is solidified. Place the coated bars on a parchment-lined tray and drizzle any remaining coating over them.

5. Refrigerate the coated bars for at least 15 minutes to harden. Keep refrigerated for up to 1 week or freeze for up to 3 months.

YIELD: 10 servings

NUTRITIONAL FACTS

Per serving (1 bar): total carbs: 5.3 g; fiber: 2.8 g; net carbs: 2.5 g; protein: 3.8 g; fat: 17.8 g; energy: 193 kcal.

Macronutrient ratio: calories from carbs: 5 percent; protein: 8 percent; fat: 87 percent.

5

SIPPABLE SNACKS:
Blissful Beverages for Any Time of Day

Low-carb snacks come in many different shapes and sizes—including refreshing smoothies and satisfying hot beverages. Plenty of the beverages in this chapter are nutritious enough to count as filling snacks. Most are high in healthy fats, which help you stay fuller longer, so they're also perfect for breakfasts or light lunches. And they're quick to prepare—most of the recipes in this chapter take only a few minutes to whip up.

Creamy Dark Hot Chocolate

Made with pure dark chocolate, coconut milk, and spices, this is the Holy Grail for low-carb chocolate fiends. Treat yourself to a (guilt-free!) cup the next time a craving strikes. (Make this nut- and dairy-free by using coconut milk and water for the first two ingredients.)

½ cup (120 ml/4 fl oz) coconut milk or heavy whipping cream

½ cup (120 ml/4 fl oz) water or almond milk

2 cardamom pods, crushed

⅛ teaspoon ground cinnamon

¼ teaspoon sugar-free vanilla extract or ⅛ teaspoon vanilla powder

Pinch salt

2 tablespoons (20 g 0.7 ounce) granulated erythritol or Swerve

1 ounce (28 g) unsweetened chocolate

1 tablespoon (15 ml/0.5 fl oz) MCT oil or coconut oil

Few drops liquid stevia, to taste (optional)

1. In a small saucepan, combine the coconut milk, water, cardamom, cinnamon, vanilla, salt, and erythritol. Bring to a boil. When bubbles form on top, remove the mixture from the heat and let it sit for 5 minutes. Add the unsweetened chocolate and MCT oil and let it melt while stirring. If you want a sweeter taste, add the stevia and stir again.

2. Pour the chocolate mixture through a sieve into a blender and pulse for a few seconds until smooth and frothy. Serve hot!

YIELD: 1 serving

....

NUTRITIONAL FACTS

Per serving: total carbs: 11.6 g; fiber: 4.2 g; net carbs: 7.4 g; protein: 6.3 g; fat: 52.9 g; energy: 528 kcal.

Macronutrient ratio: calories from carbs: 5 percent; protein: 5 percent; fat: 90 percent.

Creamy White Hot Chocolate

Never tried white hot chocolate? Now's the time! It's just as smooth and rich as its darker counterpart, and it's full of healthy fats—and it takes just five minutes to make.

½ cup (120 ml/4 fl oz) coconut milk or heavy whipping cream

½ cup (120 ml/4 fl oz) water or almond milk

¼ teaspoon sugar-free vanilla extract or ⅛ teaspoon vanilla powder

Pinch salt

1 tablespoon (10 g/0.4 oz) granulated erythritol or Swerve

1 ounce (28 g) Homemade White Chocolate (page 34)

1 tablespoon (15 ml/0.5 fl oz) MCT oil or coconut oil

Few drops liquid stevia, to taste (optional)

In a small saucepan, combine the coconut milk, water, vanilla, salt, and erythritol. Bring to a boil. When bubbles form on top, remove the mixture from the heat. Add the white chocolate and MCT oil and let it melt while stirring. If you want a sweeter taste, add the stevia and stir again. With a hand blender, pulse for a few seconds until smooth and frothy. Serve hot!

YIELD: 1 serving

....

NUTRITIONAL FACTS

Per serving: total carbs: 6.5 g fiber: 0.1 g; net carbs: 6.4 g; protein: 3 g; fat: 57.8 g; energy: 536 kcal.

Macronutrient ratio: calories from carbs: 5 percent; protein: 2 percent; fat: 93 percent.

Creamy Keto Coffee

This is an upgraded version of the popular "bulletproof" coffee, which combines butter and coconut oil for a whack of healthy fats (and an instant energy boost). Here, egg yolks—don't worry, they won't scramble—add an amazingly creamy texture and make this recipe so filling and nutritious that it can replace a regular meal. (See also Coconut-Vanilla Coffee on page 128.)

1 cup (240 ml /8 fl oz) hot brewed coffee or black tea

1 tablespoon (15 ml/0.5 fl oz) coconut milk or heavy whipping cream

1 tablespoon (15 ml/0.5 fl oz) MCT oil or coconut oil

1 tablespoon (0.5 ounce, or 14 g) unsalted butter or more coconut oil

¼ to ½ teaspoon ground cinnamon or vanilla powder

3 large egg yolks, whites reserved for another use

1 tablespoon (10 g/0.4 oz) granulated erythritol or Swerve, or 3 to 5 drops liquid stevia (optional)

In a blender, combine the coffee, coconut milk, MCT oil, butter, cinnamon, and egg yolks. Pulse until smooth and frothy. If you want a sweeter taste, add the erythritol and pulse again. Serve hot!

YIELD: 1 serving

....

NUTRITIONAL FACTS

Per serving: total carbs: 6.8 g; fiber: 0.4 g; net carbs: 6.4 g; protein: 8.8 g; fat: 42.3 g; energy: 436 kcal.

Macronutrient ratio: calories from carbs: 6 percent; protein: 8 percent; fat: 86 percent.

▶ Cutting down on caffeine? For a naturally caffeine-free alternative, try instant coffee powder made from chicory root or dandelion or make this recipe with your favorite caffeine-free tea instead.

Coconut-Vanilla Coffee

In addition to Creamy Keto Coffee (page 126), here is another version of the popular "bulletproof coffee"—coffee with unsalted butter instead of cream—only without the butter, as MCT oil is more ketogenic.

1 cup (235 ml) hot brewed coffee

1/4 cup (60 ml) unsweetened coconut milk

1 tablespoon (15 ml) MCT oil

18 drops liquid stevia (French vanilla flavor)

1/2 teaspoon vanilla extract

This is simple: Just combine everything in a blender and run until the coconut milk has melted and it's frothy.

YIELD: 1 serving

NUTRITIONAL FACTS

Per serving: total carbs: 2 g; fiber: 0 g; net carbs: 2 g; protein: 1.1 g; fat: 22.4 g; calories: 215.

Macronutrient ratio: calories from carbs: 4 percent; protein: 2 percent; fat: 92 percent.

Cococcino

Here's a frosty, sweet coffee drink for all of you who have given up dairy—and it has no sugar. Think of the money you'll save! This is perfect on a hot summer day, or anytime.

11/2 cups (355 ml) unsweetened coconut milk, chilled

2/3 cup (160 ml) brewed espresso, cooled

2 tablespoons (30 g) powdered Swerve

20 drops liquid stevia (vanilla, chocolate, hazelnut, or English toffee flavor)

About 10 ice cubes

1. Put everything but the ice in a blender and turn it on.

2. Drop in the ice cubes, one at a time, and run until the ice is pulverized. Pour and drink.

▶ **Note:** You can use sugar-free coffee-flavored syrup in place of the liquid stevia. It is less concentrated than liquid stevia; use to taste.

YIELD: 2 servings

NUTRITIONAL FACTS

Per serving (13 oz, or 366 g): total carbs: 15 g; fiber: 0 g; net carbs: 15 g; protein: 2.4 g; fat: 25.1 g; calories: 280.

Macronutrient ratio: calories from carbs: 20 percent; protein: 3 percent; fat: 77 percent.

Coconut Chai

This spiced, sweetened Indian tea is commonly made with dairy milk, but coconut milk, also popular in India, works well here, too.

8 tea bags

4 cups (950 ml) water

1/2 teaspoon liquid stevia (plain or English toffee flavor)

1 teaspoon ground cinnamon

1 teaspoon ground cardamom

1/2 teaspoon ground nutmeg

1/2 teaspoon ground ginger

1/4 teaspoon ground cloves

13/4 cups (410 ml) unsweetened coconut milk

1. In a big saucepan, combine everything but the coconut milk and bring to a boil. Turn off the burner and let it steep as it cools.

2. Strain through a fine-mesh strainer or let the spices settle to the bottom and pour off the tea as carefully as possible, leaving the powdery stuff behind.

3. Stir in the coconut milk. Store in the fridge and serve either hot or cold.

▶ **Note:** Play around with the ingredients to your liking. For instance, sub in xylitol (2 heaping tablespoons [about 18 g]) for the stevia. Use heavy cream instead of the coconut milk—for 1 cup (235 ml) chai use 1/4 cup (60 ml) cream. Optional: If using cream, make the tea ahead of time, keep it in the fridge, and then add the cream just before serving.

YIELD: 8 servings

NUTRITIONAL FACTS

Per serving (6 oz, or 168 g): total carbs: 1.4 g; fiber: 0 g; net carbs: 1.4 g; protein: 0.7 g; fat: 7.3 g; calories: 80.

Macronutrient ratio: calories from carbs: 7 percent; protein: 4 percent; fat: 89 percent.

Fat-Burning Vanilla Smoothie

You don't need to get out the frying pan to have eggs for breakfast. It's so much faster to toss them into this thick, creamy smoothie! Combined with mascarpone cheese (or creamed coconut milk for a dairy-free version) and a dash of coconut oil, it's a full meal in a glass.

2 large egg yolks, whites reserved for another use

½ cup (120 g/4.2 oz) full-fat mascarpone cheese or creamed coconut milk

¼ cup (60 ml/2 fl oz) water

4 to 5 ice cubes

1 tablespoon (15 ml/0.5 fl oz) MCT oil or coconut oil (see Note)

1 teaspoon sugar-free vanilla extract or ½ teaspoon vanilla powder

1 tablespoon (10 g/0.4 oz) erythritol or Swerve, powdered, or 3 to 5 drops liquid stevia

Whipped cream or coconut milk, for topping (optional)

If using creamed coconut milk, make it a day ahead following the instructions on page 93. In a blender, combine the egg yolks, mascarpone, water, ice, MCT oil, vanilla, and erythritol. Pulse until smooth. Top with whipped cream or coconut milk (if using).

YIELD: 1 serving

....

NUTRITIONAL FACTS

Per serving: total carbs: 4.6 g; fiber: 0.9 g; net carbs: 3.7 g; protein: 12.2 g; fat: 64.3 g; energy: 649 kcal.

Macronutrient ratio: calories from carbs: 2 percent; protein: 8 percent; fat: 90 percent.

▶ If you use coconut oil, it's important to make this using a blender to avoid leaving "pieces" of coconut oil in your smoothie. Unlike MCT oil, coconut oil is only liquid above 75°F (24°C). If you don't eat eggs, you can still enjoy this smoothie. Use 1 tablespoon (8 g/0.3 oz) of ground chia seeds or ¼ cup (25 g/0.9 oz) whey protein powder in place of the two egg yolks.

Raspberry and Vanilla Smoothie

This liquid fat bomb is another great breakfast option. It's loaded with raspberries, mascarpone, and good-for-you fats, and it's perfect for summer mornings when the weather's too warm for a hot meal.

⅓ cup (50 g/1.8 oz) raspberries, fresh or frozen

½ cup (120 g/4.2 oz) mascarpone cheese or creamed coconut milk (see page 93)

¼ cup (60 ml/2 fl oz) water

4 to 5 ice cubes

½ teaspoon sugar-free vanilla extract or ¼ teaspoon vanilla powder

1 tablespoon (15 ml/0.5 fl oz) MCT oil or coconut oil (see Note)

1 tablespoon (10 g/0.4 oz) erythritol or Swerve, powdered, or 3 to 5 drops liquid stevia (optional)

Whipped cream or coconut milk, for topping (optional)

1. If using creamed coconut milk, make it a day ahead following the instructions on page 93.

2. In a blender, combine the raspberries, mascarpone, water, ice, vanilla, and MCT oil. Pulse until smooth. If you want a sweeter taste, add the erythritol and top with whipped cream.

YIELD: 1 serving

....

NUTRITIONAL FACTS

Per serving: total carbs: 5.8 g; fiber: 1.3 g; net carbs: 4.6 g; protein: 7.5 g; fat: 55.5 g; energy: 552 kcal.

Macronutrient ratio: calories from carbs: 3 percent; protein: 6 percent; fat: 91 percent.

▶ If you use coconut oil, it's important to make this using a blender to avoid leaving "pieces" of coconut oil in your smoothie. Unlike MCT oil, coconut oil is only liquid above 75°F (24°C).

Creamy Orange Smoothie

Creamy and tangy all at once, this citrusy smoothie is as refreshing as the ice pops we loved as kids—but it's far more nutritious and filling, and, of course, it's completely sugar free.

2 large egg yolks, whites reserved for another use

½ cup (120 g/4.2 oz) full-fat mascarpone cheese or creamed coconut milk

¼ cup (60 ml/2 fl oz) water

4 to 5 ice cubes

1 tablespoon (15 ml/0.5 fl oz) MCT oil or coconut oil (see Note)

1 teaspoon freshly grated orange zest or ¼ to ½ teaspoon sugar-free orange extract

¼ teaspoon ground cinnamon

1 tablespoon (10 g/0.4 oz) erythritol or Swerve, powdered, or 3 to 5 drops liquid stevia

Whipped cream or coconut milk, for topping (optional)

1. If using creamed coconut milk, make it a day ahead following the instructions on page 93.

2. In a blender, combine the egg yolks, mascarpone, water, ice, MCT oil, orange zest, cinnamon, and erythritol. Pulse until smooth. Top with whipped cream (if using) and serve.

YIELD: 1 serving

....

NUTRITIONAL FACTS

Per serving: total carbs: 4.9 g; fiber: 0.6 g; net carbs: 4.3 g; protein: 12.3 g; fat: 64.4 g; energy: 648 kcal.

Macronutrient ratio: calories from carbs: 3 percent; protein: 7 percent; fat: 90 percent.

▶ If you use coconut oil, it's important to make this using a blender to avoid leaving "pieces" of coconut oil in your smoothie. Unlike MCT oil, coconut oil is only liquid above 75°F (24°C). If you don't eat eggs, you can still enjoy this smoothie. Use 1 tablespoon (8 g/0.3 oz) of ground chia seeds or ¼ cup (25 g/0.9 oz) whey protein powder in place of the two egg yolks.

Key Lime Smoothie

Never had avocado for breakfast before? Well, there's a first time for everything! Avocados are so nutritious, plus they're a great flavor match for lime and they add a velvety texture to this satisfying, low-carb smoothie.

½ medium (75 g/2.6 oz) ripe avocado, pitted and peeled

¼ cup (60 ml/2 fl oz) creamed coconut milk or heavy whipping cream

½ cup (120 ml/4 fl oz) water

4 to 5 ice cubes

1 tablespoon (15 ml/0.5 fl oz) MCT oil or coconut oil (see Note)

2 tablespoons (30 ml/1 fl oz) freshly squeezed lime juice

1 teaspoon freshly grated lime zest

1 tablespoon (10 g/0.4 oz) erythritol or Swerve, powdered, or 3 to 5 drops liquid stevia

Whipped cream or coconut milk, for topping (optional)

If using creamed coconut milk, make it a day ahead following the instructions on page 93. In a blender, combine the avocado, creamed coconut milk, water, ice, MCT oil, lime juice, lime zest, and erythritol. Pulse until smooth. Top with whipped cream (if using), and serve.

YIELD: 1 serving

....

NUTRITIONAL FACTS

Per serving: total carbs: 10.1 g; fiber: 5.3 g net carbs: 4.8 g; protein: 5 g; fat: 45.2 g; energy: 454 kcal.

Macronutrient ratio: calories from carbs: 4 percent; protein: 5 percent; fat: 91 percent.

▶ If you use coconut oil, it's important to make this using a blender to avoid leaving "pieces" of coconut oil in your smoothie. Unlike MCT oil, coconut oil is only liquid above 75°F (24°C).

Almond Bliss Smoothie

Chocolate, coconut, and almond—three ingredients usually found in your favorite candy bar. Transform them into a healthy smoothie with this sippable fat bomb recipe.

½ cup (120 ml/4 fl oz) coconut milk or heavy whipping cream

½ cup (120 ml/4 fl oz) almond milk

1 tablespoon (8 g/0.3 oz) chia seeds

2 tablespoons (32 g/1.1 oz) Almond Bliss Butter (page 30)

1 tablespoon (15 ml/0.5 fl oz) MCT oil or coconut oil (see Note)

1 tablespoon (10 g/0.4 oz) erythritol or Swerve, powdered, or 3 to 5 drops liquid stevia

1 teaspoon toasted, unsweetened shredded coconut or whipped cream, for topping (optional)

In a blender, combine the coconut milk, almond milk, and chia seeds. Let the mixture soak for 5 to 10 minutes. Add the Almond Bliss Butter, MCT oil, and erythritol. Pulse until smooth and creamy. Top with toasted coconut or whipped cream (if using), and serve.

YIELD: 1 serving

NUTRITIONAL FACTS

Per serving: total carbs: 13.6 g; fiber: 6.3 g; net carbs: 7.3 g; protein: 8.8 g; fat: 53.7 g; energy: 548 kcal.

Macronutrient ratio: calories from carbs: 5 percent; protein: 6 percent; fat: 89 percent.

▶ If you use coconut oil, it's important to make this using a blender to avoid leaving "pieces" of coconut oil in your smoothie. Unlike MCT oil, coconut oil is only liquid above 75°F (24°C).

Lemon Cheesecake Smoothie

Who said breakfast shouldn't taste like dessert? Not us! Satisfy your sweet tooth first thing in the morning with this scrumptious-but-sating smoothie.

¼ cup (60 g/2.1 oz) full-fat cream cheese or creamed coconut milk (see page 93)

¼ cup (60 ml/2 fl oz) heavy whipping cream or coconut milk

½ cup (120 ml/4 fl oz) water

2 tablespoons (30 ml/1 fl oz) freshly squeezed lemon juice

1 teaspoon freshly grated lemon zest

1 tablespoon (15 ml/0.5 fl oz) MCT oil or coconut oil (see Note)

1 tablespoon (10 g/0.4 oz) erythritol or Swerve, powdered, or 3 to 5 drops liquid stevia

4 to 5 ice cubes (optional)

1. If using creamed coconut milk, make it a day ahead following the instructions on page 93.

2. In a blender, combine the cream cheese, cream, water, lemon juice, lemon zest, MCT oil, and erythritol. Pulse until smooth and creamy. Serve over ice, if you like.

YIELD: 1 serving

....

NUTRITIONAL FACTS

Per serving: total carbs: 7.1 g; fiber: 1.4 g; net carbs: 5.7 g; protein: 5.5 g; fat: 52.7 g; energy: 490 kcal.

Macronutrient ratio: calories from carbs: 4 percent; protein: 4 percent; fat: 92 percent.

▶ If you use coconut oil, it's important to make this using a blender to avoid leaving "pieces" of coconut oil in your smoothie. Unlike MCT oil, coconut oil is only liquid above 75°F (24°C).

Pumpkin Pie Smoothie

Pumpkin only gets top billing in supermarket shelves in the fall—which isn't quite fair, because it's delicious year-round. It's also a great addition to just about anything, including this keto-friendly smoothie. Featured here are the homemade Pumpkin Sun Butter on page 28, sugar-free pumpkin purée, and aromatic autumnal spices.

¼ cup (60 g/2.1 oz) full-fat cream cheese or creamed coconut milk (see page 93)

¼ cup (60 ml/2 fl oz) heavy whipping cream or coconut milk

½ cup (120 ml/4 fl oz) water

1 tablespoon (16 g/0.5 oz) Pumpkin Sun Butter (page 28)

2 tablespoons (40 g/1.4 oz) unsweetened pumpkin purée

½ teaspoon pumpkin pie spice

1 tablespoon (15 ml/0.5 fl oz) MCT oil or coconut oil (see Note)

1 tablespoon (10 g/0.4 oz) erythritol or Swerve, powdered, or 3 to 5 drops liquid stevia

4 to 5 ice cubes (optional)

1. If using creamed coconut milk, make it a day ahead following the instructions on page 93.

2. In a blender, combine the cream cheese, cream, water, Pumpkin Sun Butter, pumpkin purée, pumpkin pie spice mix, MCT oil, and erythritol. Pulse until smooth and creamy. Serve over ice, if you like.

YIELD: 1 serving

....

NUTRITIONAL FACTS

Per serving: total carbs: 11.2 g; fiber: 3.3 g; net carbs: 7.9 g; protein: 9.5 g; fat: 60.7 g; energy: 587 kcal.

Macronutrient ratio: calories from carbs: 5 percent; protein: 6 percent; fat: 89 percent.

▶ If you use coconut oil, it's important to make this using a blender to avoid leaving "pieces" of coconut oil in your smoothie. Unlike MCT oil, coconut oil is only liquid above 75°F (24°C).

Chocolate-Hazelnut Smoothie

You know that sugar-laden chocolate-hazelnut spread that's so good when it's slathered on—well, just about anything? Add the homemade version in this book to a smoothie: it's even better than the store-bought stuff, and it means you get chocolate for breakfast. Don't worry—it's low carb and sugar free!

½ cup (120 ml/4 fl oz) coconut milk or heavy whipping cream

¼ cup (60 ml/2 fl oz) water

1 tablespoon (8 g/0.3 oz) chia seeds

2 tablespoons (32 g/1.1 oz) Chocolate-Hazelnut Butter (page 14)

1 tablespoon (15 ml/0.5 fl oz) MCT oil or coconut oil (see Note)

1 tablespoon (10 g/0.4 oz) erythritol or Swerve, powdered, or 3 to 5 drops liquid stevia

4 to 5 ice cubes (optional)

In a blender, combine the coconut milk, water, and chia seeds. Let the mixture soak for 5 to 10 minutes. Add the Chocolate-Hazelnut Butter, MCT oil, and erythritol. Pulse until smooth and creamy. Serve over ice, if you like.

YIELD: 1 serving

....

NUTRITIONAL FACTS

Per serving: total carbs: 12.8 g; fiber: 5.7 g; net carbs: 7.1 g; protein: 7.8 g; fat: 58.4 g; energy: 570 kcal.

Macronutrient ratio: calories from carbs: 5 percent; protein: 5 percent; fat: 90 percent.

▶ If you use coconut oil, it's important to make this using a blender to avoid leaving "pieces" of coconut oil in your smoothie. Unlike MCT oil, coconut oil is only liquid above 75°F (24°C).

6

SAFE SNACKING:
Nut-Free, Dairy-Free, and
Egg-Free Options

Welcome to an entirely nut-free chapter! Although there are nut-free recipes throughout the book, we've gathered twenty in one chapter for easy selection. Some of these recipes are also dairy-free (Sweet Bacon Kale) or egg-free (Pepperoni Pizza Fat Bombs). Many (Sweet & Salty Spiced Pepitas and Coconut Candies, among others) are all three!

Whether a food allergy affects you directly, it's likely you will face a time when you need to prepare a snack for yourself or someone who is affected, such as family, friends, or coworkers. Globally, an estimated 220 million people have food allergies, including 15 million Americans, according to End Allergies Together.

With these statistics in mind, we've made it easy so you can prepare your own safe snacks with worry-free confidence. What's more, excluding certain allergy-related foods doesn't mean you have to skimp on protein, healthy fats, or flavor. Enjoy these delicious sweet and savory snacks!

Sweet & Salty Spiced Pepitas

Pepitas are a wonderful snack because they are high in both iron and zinc, which are vital for enhancing memory, and great for strengthening your immune system and helping boost energy. Moreover, they have a perfect crunch. Add a little salt and a little sweetness and you have a fabulously addictive snack!

2 cups (450 g) raw pepitas

2 teaspoons pumpkin pie spice

1 teaspoon salt

1½ tablespoons (30 g) maple syrup

1. Preheat the oven to 350°F (180°C, or gas mark 4). Line a baking sheet with parchment paper.

2. In a medium bowl, mix together the pepitas, pumpkin pie spice, and salt. Add the maple syrup and stir until the pumpkin seed mixture is evenly coated. Spread out the seeds evenly on the prepared baking sheet and bake for 12 minutes, or until they start to turn brown, stirring halfway through so they bake evenly. Take out of the oven and allow to cool for at least 30 minutes. As they cool, they will get even crunchier! Store in an airtight container.

YIELD: 2 cups (450 g)

....

NUTRITIONAL FACTS

Per 1/4-cup serving (1⅓ oz, or 37 g): total carbs: 6.3 g; fiber: 2 g; net carbs: 4.3 g; protein: 9.8 g; fat: 15.9 g; calories: 191.

Macronutrient ratio: calories from carbs: 12 percent; protein: 19 percent; fat: 69 percent.

Sweet Bacon Kale

This easy-to-make and supertasty snack is sweet, salty, and so good you'll forget you're eating a superfood.

3 slices nitrate-free bacon, chopped into bite-size pieces

4 big handfuls kale, torn from stems

1 tablespoon (15 ml) apple cider vinegar

¼ teaspoon salt

2 or 3 drops liquid stevia

In a large skillet over medium heat, cook the bacon until brown and crispy, 8 to 10 minutes. Add the kale and cook for 5 minutes, or until the leaves soften. Mix in the vinegar, salt, and stevia. Serve immediately or save in the fridge for a snack later on.

YIELD: about 4 servings

....

NUTRITIONAL FACTS

Per serving (1 oz, or 28 g): total carbs: 1.4 g; fiber: 0.6 g; net carbs: 0.8 g; protein: 2.9 g; fat: 3.2 g; calories: 45.

Macronutrient ratio: calories from carbs: 12 percent; protein: 26 percent; fat: 62 percent.

Crispy Okra Sticks

These are a good go-to snack whenever you're in the mood for something crispy and salty. Eat them while they are fresh out of the oven and they will make traditional potato chips seem boring and bland.

½ pound (225 g) fresh okra

1 to 2 tablespoons (13.5 to 27 g) coconut

oil, melted

¼ teaspoon salt

Preheat the oven to 425°F (220°C, or gas mark 7). Rinse and dry the okra and then slice each pod in half lengthwise. Place in a mixing bowl and coat in melted coconut oil and salt. Lay the okra flat on a baking sheet (without parchment paper) and bake for 10 minutes. Turn the okra and bake for another 10 minutes, or until crispy. Serve immediately.

YIELD: about 4 servings

....

NUTRITIONAL FACTS

Per serving (2 oz, or 60 g): total carbs: 4.2 g; fiber: 1.8 g; net carbs: 2.4 g; protein: 1.1 g; fat: 3.5 g; calories: 49.

Macronutrient ratio: calories from carbs: 32 percent; protein: 8 percent; fat: 60 percent.

Pepperoni Pizza Fat Bombs

These keto-friendly fat bombs are every bit as good as delivery pepperoni pizza—minus the carb-laden crust, of course!

3.5 ounces (100 g) full-fat cream cheese, at room temperature

¼ cup (56 g/2 oz) unsalted butter, at room temperature

12 (36 g/1.3 oz) pepperoni slices

1 clove of garlic, minced

½ small red pepper (40 g/1.4 oz), finely chopped

¼ cup (28 g/1 oz) grated mozzarella cheese

1 to 2 tablespoons (5 to 10 g/0.2 to 0.4 oz) chopped fresh herbs (such as basil, oregano, thyme), or 1 to 2 teaspoons dried herbs

⅛ teaspoon chili powder

Pinch salt

½ cup (30 g/1.1 oz) grated Parmesan cheese

1. In a bowl, mash together the cream cheese and the butter with a fork, or process in a food processor until smooth.

2. In a large skillet set over medium heat, cook the pepperoni slices and on both sides until crispy. Transfer to a plate to cool.

3. Add the garlic and red pepper to the pepperoni juices in the skillet and cook for a few minutes over medium heat until fragrant. Remove from the heat and cool slightly. Add to the cream cheese and butter mixture and mix well with an electric beater or a hand whisk.

4. Add the grated mozzarella cheese, herbs, chili powder, and salt. Mix well again. Refrigerate for 20 to 30 minutes, or until set.

5. Using a large spoon or an ice cream scoop, divide the mixture into six balls. Roll each ball in the Parmesan cheese and place on top of two slices of crisped pepperoni. Enjoy immediately or refrigerate in an airtight container for up to 5 days.

YIELD: 6 servings

NUTRITIONAL FACTS

Per serving: total carbs: 1.5 g; fiber: 0.2 g; net carbs: 1.3 g; protein: 5.7 g; fat: 17.2 g; energy: 175 kcal.

Macronutrient ratio: calories from carbs: 3 percent; protein: 12 percent; fat: 85 percent.

Stilton and Chive Fat Bombs

Blue cheese addicts will adore these zero-carb fat bombs, in which pungent Stilton is suspended in a cloud of cream cheese and butter. The final flourish comes from a thorough coating of freshly chopped chives.

3.5 ounces (100 g) full-fat cream cheese, at room temperature

¼ cup (56 g/2 oz) unsalted butter, at room temperature

½ cup (65 g/2.3 oz) crumbled Stilton or other blue cheese

2 medium (30 g/1.1 oz) spring onions, finely chopped

1 tablespoon (3 g/0.1 oz) finely chopped fresh parsley

Pinch salt

⅓ cup (30 g/1.1 oz) chopped fresh chives, or more finely chopped spring onion

1. In a bowl, mash together the cream cheese and butter, or process in a food processor until smooth.

2. Add the crumbled Stilton, spring onions, and parsley. Mix until well combined. Season with salt. Refrigerate for 20 to 30 minutes, or until set.

3. Using a large spoon or an ice cream scoop, divide the mixture into six balls. Roll each ball in the chopped chives and place on a plate. Enjoy immediately or refrigerate in an airtight container for up to 5 days.

YIELD: 6 servings

NUTRITIONAL FACTS

Per serving: total carbs: 1.1 g; fiber: 0.2 g; net carbs: 0.8 g; protein: 4.5 g; fat: 16.2 g; energy: 157 kcal.

Macronutrient ratio: calories from carbs: 2 percent; protein: 11 percent; fat: 87 percent.

Bacon and Guacamole Fat Bombs

There's only one way to improve upon homemade guacamole, and that's to transform it into bacon-coated fat bombs. Seriously.

4 large bacon slices (120 g /4.2 oz)

½ large (100 g /3.5 oz) avocado, halved, pitted, and peeled

¼ cup (56 g /2 oz) unsalted butter or ghee, at room temperature

2 garlic cloves, crushed

1 small chile pepper, finely chopped

1 tablespoon (15 ml/0.5 fl oz) fresh lime juice

Salt and pepper, to taste

½ small (35 g /1.2 oz) white onion, diced

1. Preheat the oven to 375°F (/190°C, or gas mark 5). Line a rimmed baking sheet with parchment paper. Be sure to use a rimmed sheet to contain the bacon fat, as you'll need it for the recipe, too. Lay the bacon strips flat on the parchment, leaving enough space between so they don't overlap. Place the sheet in the preheated oven and cook for 10 to 15 minutes, or until crispy. The exact amount of cooking time depends on the thickness of the bacon slices. Remove from the oven and set aside to cool. When cool enough to handle, crumble the bacon into a bowl and set aside.

2. In a bowl, combine the avocado, butter, garlic, chile pepper, and lime juice. Season with salt and pepper. Mash with a potato masher or fork until well combined. Stir in the onion. Pour in the bacon grease from the baking sheet and mix well. Cover with aluminum foil and refrigerate for 20 to 30 minutes.

3. Using a large spoon or an ice cream scoop, divide the mixture into 6 balls. If serving immediately, roll them in the crumbled bacon. If serving later, re-frigerate without the bacon coating in an airtight container for up to 5 days. Roll the fat bombs in freshly cooked or reheated bacon crumbs just before serving.

YIELD: 6 servings

....

NUTRITIONAL FACTS

Per serving: total carbs: 2.7 g; fiber: 1.3 g; net carbs: 1.4 g; protein: 3.4 g; fat: 15.2 g; energy: 156 kcal.

Macronutrient ratio: calories from carbs: 3 percent; protein: 9 percent; fat: 88 percent.

Ham and Cheese Fat Bombs

There are few things that can't be improved by a cloak of sweet-and-salty Parma ham—and these creamy, basil-flecked fat bombs are no exception. Try them as a low-carb afternoon snack.

3.5 ounces (100 g) full-fat cream cheese, at room temperature

¼ cup (56 g/2 oz) unsalted butter, at room temperature

¼ cup (30 g/1.1 oz) grated Cheddar or Gouda cheese

2 tablespoons (10 g/0.4 oz) chopped fresh basil

Salt and pepper, to taste

6 slices (90 g/3.2 oz) Parma ham

6 large (30 g/1.1 oz) green olives, pitted

1. In a bowl, mash together the cream cheese and butter, or process in a food processor until smooth.

2. Add the Cheddar and basil and mix until well combined. Season with salt and pepper. Refrigerate for 20 to 30 minutes, or until set.

3. Using a large spoon or an ice-cream scoop, divide the mixture into six balls. Wrap each ball in one slice of Parma ham and place on a plate. Top each ball with one olive and pierce with a toothpick to hold it in place. Enjoy immediately or refrigerate in an airtight container for up to 5 days.

YIELD: 6 servings

....

NUTRITIONAL FACTS

Per serving: total carbs: 0.9 g; fiber: 0.2 g; net carbs: 0.7 g; protein: 6.4 g; fat: 16.4 g; energy: 167 kcal.

Macronutrient ratio: calories from carbs: 2 percent; protein: 14 percent; fat: 84 percent.

Veggie and Cheese Fat Bombs

Just like a gourmet vegetable pizza only sans *carbs, these tasty fat bombs feature caramelized onion, porcini mushrooms, fresh spinach, and goat cheese.*

3.5 ounces (100 g) full-fat cream cheese, at room temperature

1/4 cup (56 g/2 oz) unsalted butter, at room temperature

1 tablespoon (15 g/0.5 oz) ghee

1/2 small (35 g/1.2 oz) white onion, peeled and finely chopped

1 clove of garlic, peeled and finely chopped

1/2 cup (15 g/0.5 oz) dried porcini mushrooms, soaked in 1 cup (235 ml) warm water for 30 minutes and then drained and sliced

2 cups (60 g/2.1 oz) fresh spinach

Salt and pepper, to taste

1/4 cup (30 g/2.1 oz) grated hard goat cheese

1. In a bowl, mash together the cream cheese and butter, or process in a food processor until smooth.

2. Grease a hot pan with the ghee. Add the onion and garlic and cook over medium heat for 2 to 3 minutes, or until fragrant. Add the mushrooms and cook for about 2 minutes more. Add the spinach and cook for 1 minute more, or until wilted. Remove the pan from the heat and set aside to cool.

3. Add the cooled mushroom and spinach mixture to the cream cheese and butter and mix until well combined. Season with salt and pepper. Refrigerate for 20 to 30 minutes, or until set.

4. Using a large spoon or an ice cream scoop, divide the mixture into six balls. Roll each ball in the goat cheese. Enjoy immediately or refrigerate in an airtight container for up to 5 days.

YIELD: 6 servings

NUTRITIONAL FACTS

Per serving: total carbs: 3.6 g; fiber: 0.6 g; net carbs: 3 g; protein: 3.4 g; fat: 16.7 g; energy: 166 kcal.

Macronutrient ratio: calories from carbs: 7 percent; protein: 8 percent; fat: 85 percent.

Smoked Mackerel Pâté Fat Bombs

If you're a fan of smoked fish, you're sure to love this low-carb dip. It's lightened and brightened by a dash of fresh lime juice and a handful of chives.

3.5 ounces (100 g) full-fat cream cheese, at room temperature

¼ cup (56 g/2 oz) unsalted butter, at room temperature

1 medium (100 g/3.5 oz) smoked mackerel fillet

1 tablespoon (15 ml/0.5 fl oz) freshly squeezed lime juice

2 tablespoons (8 g/0.3 oz) chopped fresh chives

Cucumber slices, for serving (optional)

In a food processor, combine the cream cheese, butter, mackerel, and lime juice. Pulse until smooth. Transfer to a bowl, add the chives, and mix with a spoon. Refrigerate for 20 to 30 minutes, or until set. Enjoy as a dip with cucumber slices, or refrigerate in an airtight container for up to 1 week.

YIELD: 6 servings

NUTRITIONAL FACTS

Per serving: total carbs: 0.8 g; fiber: 0.1 g; net carbs: 0.7 g; protein: 4.9 g; fat: 16.5 g; energy: 161 kcal.

Macronutrient ratio: calories from carbs: 2 percent; protein: 11 percent; fat: 87 percent.

Earl Grey Truffles

Earl Grey tea adds a haunting, delicate flavor to these dark chocolate truffles. Be sure to use high-quality tea: it really does yield a better result.

FOR TRUFFLES:

2/3 cup (150 ml /5 fl oz) coconut milk or heavy whipping cream

1/2 cup (80 g/2.8 oz) powdered erythritol or Swerve

1/4 cup (2 ounces, or 56 g) unsalted butter, ghee, or coconut oil, at room temperature

1 tablespoon (5 g/0.2 oz) good-quality earl grey tea leaves

6 ounces (170 g) unsweetened chocolate, broken into small pieces

Pinch salt

Few drops liquid stevia, to taste (optional)

1 tablespoon (14 g/0.5 oz) macadamia oil or other light-tasting oil, for shaping the truffles

FOR COATING:

4.2 ounces (120 g) Homemade White Chocolate (page 34)

2 tablespoons (28 g/1 oz) cacao nibs

1. To make the truffles: In a saucepan, combine the coconut milk, erythritol, and butter. Bring to a boil. Immediately remove the mixture from the heat and stir in the tea. Cover and let sit for 5 to 10 minutes.

2. In a bowl, place the unsweetened chocolate piece. Through a sieve, slowly pour the hot coconut milk over the chocolate, pressing on the tea leaves as the sieve catches them. Discard the tea leaves. Stir until the chocolate is completely melted and smooth. If the chocolate mixture separates, add a splash of boiling water or place in a blender and process until smooth. Add the salt. If you want a sweeter taste, add the stevia. Cool and refrigerate for 1 hour, or until firm.

3. To shape the truffles, dip a spoon or melon baller in warm water and scoop out fourteen balls of the chilled mixture. Lightly coat your hands in maca-damia oil. Roll the truffles between your palms to form spheres about twice the size of "standard" truffles. Place on a parchment-lined tray and freeze for about 30 minutes.

4. To make the coating: Melt the white chocolate in a double boiler, or heat-proof bowl placed over a small saucepan filled with 1 cup of water, over medium heat. Once melted, remove from the heat and set aside to cool.

5. Gently pierce each frozen truffle with a toothpick or a fork. Working one at a time, hold each truffle over the melted white chocolate and spoon the chocolate over it to coat completely. Turn the stick as you work until the coating is solidified. Place the coated truffles on a parchment-lined tray and drizzle any remaining coating over them. Before the truffles become completely solid, sprinkle them with the cacao nibs.

6. Refrigerate the coated truffles for at least 15 minutes to harden. Keep refrigerated for up to 1 week or freeze for up to 3 months.

YIELD: 14 servings

NUTRITIONAL FACTS

Per serving (1 truffle): total carbs: 5.1 g; fiber: 2 g; net carbs: 3.1 g; protein: 2.5 g; fat: 20.1 g; energy: 208 kcal.

Macronutrient ratio: calories from carbs: 6 percent; protein: 5 percent; fat: 89 percent.

Toasted Coconut Cups

These cups are surprisingly easy to make! Toasting the coconut brings out its natural sweetness and adds some crunch.

1½ cups (112 g/4 oz) unsweetened desiccated, shredded, or flaked coconut

¼ cup (55 g/1.9 oz) extra virgin coconut oil, at room temperature

¼ cup (56 g/2 oz) unsalted butter, or more coconut oil, at room temperature

¼ teaspoon ground cinnamon or vanilla powder

Pinch salt

Few drops liquid stevia, to taste, or 2 tablespoons (0.7 ounce, or 20 g) erythritol or Swerve, powdered (optional)

1. Preheat the oven to 350°F (175°C, or gas mark 4). Spread the coconut on a baking sheet. Place it in the oven and toast for 5 to 8 minutes, or until lightly golden. Stir once or twice to prevent burning. Remove from the oven and cool for 5 minutes. Transfer to a food processor and pulse until smooth. This may take time. At first, the mixture will be dry. Scrape down the sides of your processor several times with a rubber spatula if the mixture sticks. The final consistency should be smooth and runny.

2. Add the coconut oil. Then add the butter, 2 tablespoons (28 g) at a time, pulsing after each addition. Add the cinnamon and salt. Pulse to mix well. If you want a sweeter taste, add the stevia and pulse again.

3. Fill a mini muffin tin or ice cube tray with 2 tablespoon (20 g/0.7 oz) portions. It should yield twelve servings. Refrigerate for at least 30 minutes, or until solid. Keep refrigerated for up to 1 week, as the coconut oil and butter become very soft at room temperature, or freeze for up to 3 months.

YIELD: 12 servings

....

NUTRITIONAL FACTS

Per serving (1 fat bomb): total carbs: 2.6 g; fiber: 1.9 g; net carbs: 0.7 g; protein: 1.9 g; fat: 9.6 g; energy: 104 kcal.

Macronutrient ratio: calories from carbs: 3 percent; protein: 8 percent; fat: 89 percent.

Chewy Hempseed Squares

Hempseeds are low in carbohydrates and high in protein and healthy fats, so they're perfect for making nut-free fat bombs. These sweet, sugar-free squares are bound with homemade condensed milk and framed by thin layers of chocolate.

FOR SQUARES:

1 can (400 ml/13.5 fl oz) coconut milk or equivalent amount of heavy whipping cream

1/4 cup (40 g/1.4 oz) erythritol or Swerve, powdered

2 teaspoons sugar-free vanilla extract or 1 teaspoon vanilla powder

1 teaspoon ground cinnamon

1/4 cup (55 g/1.9 oz) coconut oil

2 tablespoons (16 g/0.6 oz) ground chia seeds

1 1/2 cups (210 g/7.4 oz) hemp seeds, hulled

Few drops liquid stevia, to taste (optional)

FOR COATING:

7.1 ounces (200 g) Homemade Dark Chocolate (page 32)

1. To make the squares: In a small saucepan set over medium heat, bring the coconut milk to a boil. Once simmering, reduce the heat to low. Stir in the erythritol, vanilla, and cinnamon, stirring until the erythritol is dissolved. Cook for 20 to 30 minutes, stirring occasionally, until the milk is creamy and reduced by about half. Remove from the heat and mix in the coconut oil, chia seeds, and hempseeds. If you want a sweeter taste, add the stevia and mix again. Let the mixture sit for 5 to 10 minutes and then refrigerate for about 30 minutes.

2. To make the coating: Melt the dark chocolate in a double boiler, or heat-proof bowl placed over a small saucepan filled with 1 cup (235 ml) of water, over medium heat. Pour half into an 8 x 8 inch (20 x 20 cm) parchment-lined pan, or a silicone pan. With a spatula, spread the chocolate over the bottom of the pan. Refrigerate for about 15 minutes, or until hardened. Reserve the other half of the melted chocolate for the topping.

3. Remove both the chocolate and hempseed mixtures from the refrigerator. With a spatula, spread and flatten the hempseed mixture over the chilled chocolate mixture. Top with the remaining melted chocolate. Refrigerate for 45 to 60 minutes to set before slicing. Keep refrigerated for up to 1 week or freeze for up to 3 months.

YIELD: 16 servings

....
NUTRITIONAL FACTS

Per serving (1 square): total carbs: 4.4 g; fiber: 2.2 g; net carbs: 2.2 g; protein: 5.8 g; fat: 22.9 g; energy: 231 kcal.

Macronutrient ratio: calories from carbs: 4 percent; protein: 9 percent; fat: 87 percent.

▶ **Note:** Nutritional Facts are calculated using Homemade Dark Chocolate made with coconut oil (see recipe on page 32).

Chocolate-Avocado Truffles

Avocado doesn't turn up in desserts as often as it should because it's high in healthy fats and potassium—and its neutral taste and creamy texture make it a handy tool for creating decadent, low-carb chocolate truffles!

FOR TRUFFLES:

3.5 ounces (100 g) dark chocolate, 90 percent cacao solids or more, or use any of the Homemade Dark Chocolate recipes (page 32)

1 medium (150 g/5.3 oz) avocado, peeled and pitted

¼ cup (60 g/2.1 oz) coconut butter

1 teaspoon sugar-free vanilla extract or ½ teaspoon vanilla powder

½ teaspoon ground cinnamon

Pinch salt

Few drops liquid stevia, to taste (optional)

1 tablespoon (14 g/0.5 oz) macadamia oil or avocado oil, or other light-tasting oil, for shaping the truffles

FOR COATING:

2 tablespoons (10 g/0.4 oz) unsweetened cacao powder, or enough toasted almond flakes, shredded unsweetened coconut, or coconut flakes to cover

1. To make the truffles: Melt the dark chocolate in a double boiler, or heat-proof bowl placed over a small saucepan filled with 1 cup (235 ml) of water, over medium heat. Remove from heat and set aside.

2. In a food processor, combine the avocado, coconut butter, vanilla, cinnamon, and salt. Pulse until smooth. With the processor running, slowly drizzle in the melted chocolate. Mix until well combined with the avocado. If you want a sweeter taste, add the stevia. Transfer the mixture to a bowl and refrigerate for about 1 hour, or until solid.

3. To shape the truffles, dip a spoon or a melon baller in warm water and scoop out ten balls of the chilled mixture. Lightly coat your hands in macadamia oil. Roll the truffles between your palms to form spheres about twice the size of "standard" truffles. Coat them immediately after shaping.

4. To make the coating: Roll the truffles in your favorite coating. Refrigerate the coated truffles for at least 15 minutes to harden. Keep refrigerated for up to 1 week or freeze for up to 3 months.

YIELD: 10 servings

NUTRITIONAL FACTS

Per serving (1 truffle): total carbs: 5.3 g; fiber: 3 g; net carbs: 2.3 g; protein: 1.9 g; fat: 12.7 g; energy: 129 kcal.

Macronutrient ratio: calories from carbs: 7 percent; protein: 6 percent; fat: 87 percent.

Chocolate Chia Workout Bars

Often referred to as a "superfood" for good reason, chia seeds are a fantastic source of energy for a workout. They digest easily and are absorbed quickly. Just a few bites of these tasty bars will give you a boost of power and keep you sustained for the duration of your activity. Be forewarned: You might not want to eat these too late in the day as the cacao powder might give you too much energy!

1 cup (220 g) coconut butter

⅓ cup (115 g) dark raw honey

½ cup (113 g) salted and roasted sunflower seeds

½ cup (82 g) chia seeds

⅓ cup (27 g) raw cacao powder

¼ cup (20 g) unsweetened shredded coconut

¼ cup (44 g) dark chocolate chips

¼ teaspoon salt

In a small saucepan over low heat, melt the coconut butter and honey. While that is warming up, in a medium bowl, mix together the sunflower seeds, chia seeds, cacao powder, coconut, chocolate chips, and salt. When the liquids are melted, after about 5 minutes, pour them over the dry ingredients and stir well. Pour the mixture onto a baking sheet lined with parchment paper. Use another piece of parchment paper to flatten the mixture to about ¼ inch (6.5 mm) thick and then refrigerate for 1 hour. Once it has solidified, cut into bars. Store in the fridge or freezer.

YIELD: about 12 bars

....

NUTRITIONAL FACTS

Per bar: total carbs: 21.9 g; fiber: 5.8 g; net carbs: 15.8 g; protein: 4 g; fat: 21.4 g; calories: 295.

Macronutrient ratio: calories from carbs: 30 percent; protein: 5 percent; fat: 65 percent.

Cinnamon Donut Holes

Donuts are hard to re-create in low-carb form because of the texture and ingredients. Needless to say, these taste like, and have the texture of, a real donut!

½ cup (56 g) coconut flour

2 tablespoons (16 g) psyllium husk powder

¼ cup (48 g) coconut palm sugar, plus 2 tablespoons (24 g) for dipping

¼ teaspoon salt

1 cup (235 ml) water

¼ cup (55 g) grass-fed butter, plus 2 tablespoons (28 g) for dipping (can omit to make dairy-free)

1 tablespoon (7 g) ground cinnamon

1. Preheat the oven 325°F (170°C, or gas mark 3). Line a baking sheet with parchment paper.

2. In a medium bowl, mix together the coconut flour, psyllium husk powder, ¼ cup (48 g) coconut palm sugar, and salt. In a small pot, boil the water, turn off stove and then add ¼ cup (55 g) butter and stir until the butter is melted. Add the wet ingredients to the dry. When the mixture has cooled enough for you to handle, squish the dough together until it forms a firm ball.

3. Tear off golf ball–size pieces of dough and form them into donut holes. Place the balls on the prepared baking sheet. Melt the remaining 2 tablespoons (28 g) butter in a small bowl. In another small bowl, mix together 2 table-spoons (24 g) coconut palm sugar and 1 tablespoon cinnamon. Take each donut hole dough ball and dip it in the butter, making sure to coat it all over. Then, roll it into the sugar-cinnamon mixture. Place it back on the baking sheet and repeat until you have covered all of the balls of dough. Bake about 25 minutes or until a toothpick inserted in the middle comes out clean. Eat them while they are warm!

4. Alternatively (or in addition to), if you don't want to use cinnamon, you could melt some dark chocolate and drizzle it over the donut holes once they come out of the oven. Mmmmm.

YIELD: About 12 donut holes

NUTRITIONAL FACTS

Per donut: total carbs: 9.5 g; fiber: 3.3 g; net carbs: 6.2 g; protein: 0.7 g; fat: 5.2 g; calories: 85.

Macronutrient ratio: calories from carbs: 44 percent; protein: 3 percent; fat: 53 percent.

Minty Thins

Year after year, the Girl Scouts' Thin Mint cookies bring in the most sales. And it's no wonder why, with their crispy texture and sweet minty flavor. Unfortunately, with hydrogenated oil and unhealthy preservatives, Thin Mints are a cookie we can live without. Fortunately, with this recipe, we don't have to miss them. These are so good, it's hard to tell them apart from the originals, except you'll feel much better after eating these.

½ cup (112 g) plus 3 tablespoons (45 g) grass-fed butter, melted and divided

¼ cup (85 g) maple syrup

¼ cup (20 g) raw cacao powder

1 teaspoon baking soda

1 teaspoon peppermint extract

1 egg

¾ cup (84 g) coconut flour

1½ cups (263 g) dark chocolate chips

1. In a medium bowl, blend together ½ cup (112 g) butter, maple syrup, cacao powder, baking soda, and peppermint extract with a hand mixer or a whisk. In a small bowl, beat the egg and then add it to the butter-syrup mixture. Mix well until it forms a soft batter. Mix in the coconut flour in small increments until well combined. On parchment paper, hand roll the dough into a long cylinder 2½ to 3 inches (6.5 to 7.5 cm)-thick and refrigerate for 30 minutes.

2. Preheat the oven to 350°F (180°C, or gas mark 4). Once the dough has hardened, slice the dough into ¼ inch (6.5 mm) rounds and place them onto a baking sheet lined with parchment paper. Bake for 7 to 9 minutes, or until set, and then allow to cool for 30 minutes. You can put the baking sheet in the fridge to speed up the process.

3. In a heat-safe bowl, add the chocolate chips and remaining 3 tablespoons (45 g) butter and set the bowl over a saucepan of simmering water to let the chocolate and butter melt. Before the chocolate is completely melted, remove the bowl from heat and stir the chocolate until it is smooth. Allow the chocolate to cool for about 10 minutes so you don't burn yourself. Once it is cool enough, using your hands, dip each cookie and cover it completely with chocolate (it will get a little messy) and then place the cookie on the parchment paper. Once you finish coating all of the cookies, place the baking sheet in the fridge so they can cool and harden. Store them in a sealed container in the fridge or freezer.

YIELD: 36 cookies

....

NUTRITIONAL FACTS

Per cookie: total carbs: 9.2 g; fiber: 0.8 g; net carbs: 7.7 g; protein: 1.2 g; fat: 7.2 g; calories: 99

Macronutrient ratio: calories from carbs: 35 percent; protein: 5 percent; fat: 61 percent.

Red Velvet Truffles

There's no need to rely on artificial food coloring to make these beautiful truffles. Instead, use beetroot powder to give them a vivid, deep red tint.

FOR TRUFFLES:

½ cup (125 g/4.4 oz) coconut butter

¼ cup (55 g/1.9 oz) coconut oil

½ cup (60 g/2.1 oz) coconut flour

¼ cup (40 g/1.4 oz) erythritol or Swerve, powdered

2 teaspoons sugar-free vanilla extract or 1 teaspoon vanilla powder, or use the same amount of any food extract: cherry and raspberry work well

2 tablespoons (12 g/0.4 oz) beetroot powder

Pinch salt

Few drops liquid stevia, to taste (optional)

1 tablespoon (14 g/0.5 oz) macadamia oil, or other light tasting oil, for shaping the truffles

FOR COATING:

3.5 ounces (100 g) Homemade White Chocolate (page 34)

1. To make the truffles: Melt the coconut butter and coconut oil in a double boiler, or heat-proof bowl placed over a small saucepan filled with 1 cup of water, over medium heat. Remove from the heat and set aside. Stir in the coconut flour, erythritol, vanilla, beetroot powder, and salt. If you want a sweeter taste, add the stevia and mix again. Refrigerate the mixture for about 30 minutes, or until just firm enough to form truffles.

2. To shape the truffles, dip a spoon or a melon baller in warm water and scoop out ten balls of the chilled mixture. Lightly coat your hands in macadamia oil. Roll the truffles between your palms to form spheres about twice the size of "standard" truffles. Place the truffles on a parchment-lined tray. Freeze for about 30 minutes.

3. To make the coating: Melt the white chocolate in a double boiler, or heat-proof bowl placed over a small saucepan filled with 1 cup (235 ml) of water, over medium heat. Remove from the heat and set aside to cool. The chocolate should not be hot when you use it for coating.

4. Gently pierce each frozen truffle with a toothpick or a fork. Working one at a time, hold each truffle over the melted white chocolate and spoon the chocolate over it to coat completely. Turn the stick as you work until the coating is

solidified. Place the coated truffles on a parchment-lined tray and drizzle any remaining coating over them.

5. Refrigerate the coated truffles for at least 15 minutes to harden. Keep refrigerated for up to 1 month or freeze for up to 3 months.

YIELD: 10 servings

....

NUTRITIONAL FACTS

Per serving (1 truffle): total carbs: 6.5 g; fiber: 3.2 g; net carbs: 3.3 g; protein: 2.2 g; fat: 21.7 g; energy: 225 kcal.

Macronutrient ratio: calories from carbs: 6 percent; protein: 4 percent; fat: 90 percent.

Coconut Candies

Sweets don't have to be high in carbs. These versatile candies can be made with your favorite flavors—and, happily, they won't spike your blood sugar.

FOR CANDIES:

½ cup (125 g/4.4 oz) coconut butter, at room temperature

½ cup (110 g/3.9 oz) coconut oil, at room temperature

¼ cup (40 g/1.4 oz) erythritol or Swerve, powdered

1 teaspoon sugar-free extract of your choice (such as vanilla, lemon, peppermint, or almond)

Few drops liquid stevia, to taste (optional)

FOR COATING (or use any Homemade Dark Chocolate recipe [page 32]):

3 ounces (85 g) extra-dark 90 percent chocolate

1.2 ounces (35 g) cacao butter

1. To make the candies: In a bowl, combine the coconut butter, coconut oil, erythritol, and flavoring extract. Mix until well combined. If you want a sweeter taste, add the stevia.

2. Fill a silicone candy mold, silicone ice-cube trays, or mini muffin cups with about 1 tablespoon (15 g) portions of the coconut mixture. Freeze for 30 minutes to 1 hour.

3. To make the coating: Melt the dark chocolate and cacao butter in a double boiler, or heat-proof bowl placed over a small saucepan filled with 1 cup (235 ml) of water, over medium heat. Mix well. Let the chocolate cool before use. It shouldn't be hot, but should still be liquid. If you are using any of the Homemade Dark Chocolate recipes (page 32), you may need as much as 5.3 to 5.6 ounces (150 to 160 g) to coat all the fat bombs.

4. Gently pierce each frozen candy with a toothpick or a fork. Working one at a time, hold each candy over the melted chocolate and spoon the chocolate over it to coat completely. Turn the stick as you work until the coating is solidified. Place the candies on a parchment-lined tray and drizzle any remaining chocolate over them.

5. Refrigerate the coated candies for at least 15 minutes to harden. Keep refrigerated for up to 1 month or freeze for up to 3 months.

YIELD: 10 servings

....
NUTRITIONAL FACTS

Per serving (1 candy): total carbs: 2.3 g; fiber: 1.2 g; net carbs: 1 g; protein: 0.8 g; fat: 13.1 g; energy: 123 kcal.

Macronutrient ratio: calories from carbs: 3 percent; protein: 3 percent; fat: 94 percent.

Pumpkin-Snickerdoodle Truffles

Indulge your pumpkin pie cravings this fall with these pumpkin-flavored truffles! These sugar-free fat bombs are finished with a quick roll in a sweet, cinnamon-spiced coating.

FOR TRUFFLES:

½ cup (125 g/4.4 oz) coconut butter

¼ cup (55 g/2 oz) coconut oil

½ cup (100 g/3.5 oz) unsweetened pumpkin purée

2 teaspoons pumpkin pie spice

1 teaspoon sugar-free vanilla extract or ½ teaspoon vanilla powder

2 tablespoons (20 g/0.7 oz) erythritol or Swerve, powdered

2 heaping tablespoons (24 g/0.8 oz) coconut flour

Pinch salt

Few drops liquid stevia, to taste (optional)

1 tablespoon (14 g/0.5 oz) macadamia oil or other light-tasting oil, for shaping the truffles

FOR COATING:

2 tablespoons (20 g/0.7 oz) erythritol or Swerve, powdered

1½ teaspoons ground cinnamon

1. To make the truffles: Melt the coconut butter and coconut oil in a double boiler, or heat-proof bowl placed over a small saucepan filled with 1 cup (235 ml) of water, over medium heat. Remove from the heat and set aside.

2. Stir in the pumpkin purée, pumpkin pie spice mix, vanilla, erythritol, coconut flour, and salt, until combined well. If you want a sweeter taste, add the stevia. Refrigerate for 30 minutes to 1 hour, or until firm enough to form truffles.

3. To shape the truffles, dip a spoon or melon baller in warm water and scoop out ten balls of the chilled mixture. Lightly coat your hands in macadamia oil. Roll the truffles between your palms to form spheres about twice the size of "standard" truffles. Coat the truffles immediately after shaping.

4. To make the coating: In a bowl, mix together the erythritol and cinnamon. Roll the truffles in the cinnamon mixture. Refrigerate the coated truffles for at least 15 minutes to harden. Keep in the refrigerator for up to 1 week or freeze for up to 3 months.

YIELD: 10 servings

NUTRITIONAL FACTS

Per serving (1 truffle): total carbs: 5 g; fiber: 3 g; net carbs: 2 g; protein: 1.3 g; fat: 12.7 g; energy: 132 kcal.

Macronutrient ratio: calories from carbs: 6 percent; protein: 4 percent; fat: 90 percent.

Creamy Orange Ice Bombs

Bind the warm, seductive flavors of cinnamon and orange with mascarpone and cream, then ice them and coat them with coconut butter. The result? A wonderfully refreshing sugar-free snack.

FOR ICE BOMBS:

1 cup (240 g/8.5 oz) full-fat mascarpone cheese or creamed coconut milk

¼ cup (60 ml/2 fl oz) heavy whipping cream

¼ cup (40 g/1.4 oz) erythritol or Swerve, powdered

1 tablespoon (6 g/0.2 oz) freshly grated orange zest or 1 to 2 teaspoons sugar-free orange extract

¼ teaspoon ground cinnamon

Few drops liquid stevia, to taste (optional)

FOR COATING:

⅔ cup (160 g/5.6 oz) coconut butter

2 tablespoons (28 g/1 oz) coconut oil

1 teaspoon freshly grated orange zest

Pinch ground cinnamon

1. If using creamed coconut milk, make it following the instructions on page 93.

2. To make the ice bombs: In a food processor or with a mixer, combine the mascarpone, cream, erythritol, orange zest, and cinnamon. Pulse until smooth and creamy. If you want a sweeter taste, add the stevia and pulse again.

3. Spoon about 2 tablespoons (30 g/1.1 oz) of the mixture into each of twelve small silicone muffin molds or candy molds, or use round cake pop molds for a round bomb shape. Freeze for about 2 hours, or until set.

4. To make the coating: Melt together the coconut butter, coconut oil, orange zest, and cinnamon in a double boiler, or heat-proof bowl placed over a small saucepan filled with 1 cup (235 ml) of water, over medium heat. Cool before use. It should not be hot, but should still be liquid.

5. Work in batches of three or four to prevent the ice bombs from melting. Gently pierce each frozen ice bomb with a toothpick or a fork. One at a time, hold each ice bomb over the coconut mixture and spoon the mixture over it to coat completely. Turn the stick as you work until the coating is solidified. Place the coated ice bombs on a parchment-lined.

6. Freeze the coated pieces, in batches as you work, for at least 15 minutes to harden. Keep frozen for up to 3 months.

YIELD: 12 servings

....

NUTRITIONAL FACTS

Per serving (1 ice bomb): total carbs: 3.1 g; fiber: 1.8 g; net carbs: 1.3 g; protein: 1.8 g; fat: 15.9 g; energy: 158 kcal.

Macronutrient ratio: calories from carbs: 3 percent; protein: 5 percent; fat: 92 percent.

About the Authors

MARTINA SLAJEROVA is a health and food blogger living in the United Kingdom. She holds a degree in economics and worked in auditing, but has always been passionate about nutrition and healthy living. Martina loves food, science, photography, and creating new recipes. She is a firm believer in low-carb living and regular exercise. As a science geek, she bases her views on valid research and has firsthand experience of what it means to be on a low-carb diet. Both are reflected on her blog, in her KetoDiet apps, and this book.

The KetoDiet is an ongoing project she started with her partner in 2012 and includes The KetoDiet Cookbook, Fat Bombs, and the KetoDiet apps for the iPad and iPhone (www.ketodietapp.com). When creating recipes, she doesn't focus on just the carb content: You won't find any processed foods, unhealthy vegetable oils, or artificial sweeteners in her recipes.

This book and the KetoDiet apps are for people who follow a healthy low-carb lifestyle. Martina's mission is to help you reach your goals, whether it's your dream weight or simply eating healthy food. You can find even more low-carb recipes, diet plans, and information about the keto diet on her blog: www.ketodietapp.com/blog.

LANDRIA VOIGT, C.H.H.C., is a nutritional consultant and public speaker. In her twenties, she was diagnosed with an autoimmune disease and for years struggled to keep flares in check with traditional, conventional approaches. After more than a decade of suffering and frustration, she took her health into her own hands, casting aside the drugs and carefully experimenting with her own diet. The results were nothing short of miraculous.

As a result of her journey, she came to appreciate the power of nutrition and how challenging it can be to separate facts from dubious marketing spin when choosing the right foods for one's self and family. Now she is on a mission to help others enjoy healthier living through informed eating. Through public speaking engagements and consulting at The Atlanta Center for Holistic and Integrative Medicine for Taz "Dr. Taz" Bhatia, M.D., patients in Atlanta, she shares her knowledge and most up-to-date research on the ever changing subjects of food and wellness.

Through her blog stiritup.me, Landria shares her healthy recipes aimed at pleasing even the most finicky of palates, as well as forward-thinking ideas about nutrition.

In retrospect, **DANA CARPENDER'S** career seems inevitable: She's been cooking since she had to stand on a step stool to reach the stove. She was also a dangerously sugar-addicted child, eventually stealing from her parents to support her habit, and was in Weight Watchers by age eleven. At nineteen, Dana read her first book on nutrition and recognized herself in a list of symptoms of reactive hypoglycemia. She ditched sugar and white flour, and was dazzled by the near-instantaneous improvement in her physical and mental health. A lifetime nutrition buff was born.

Unfortunately, in the late eighties and early nineties, Dana got sucked into low-fat/high-carb mania, and whole-grain-and-beaned her way up to a size 20, with nasty energy swings, constant hunger, and borderline high blood pressure. In 1995, she read a nutrition book from the 1950s that stated that obesity had nothing to do with how much one ate, but was rather a carbohydrate intolerance disease. She thought, "What the heck, might as well give it a try." Three days later, her clothes were loose, her hunger was gone, and her energy level was through the roof. She never looked back, and has now been low carb for nineteen years and counting—a third of her life.

Realizing that this change was permanent, and being a cook at heart, Dana set about creating as varied and satisfying a cuisine as she could with a minimal carb load. And being an enthusiastic, gregarious sort, she started sharing her experience. By 1997 she was writing about it. The upshot is more than 2,500 recipes published, and over a million books sold—and she still has ideas left to try!

Dana lives in Bloomington, Indiana, with her husband, three dogs, and a cat, all of whom are well and healthily fed.

Index